"Brianne has a gift for understanding the female body and explaining it in a kind and easy to understand way. *Lady Bits* provides practical steps to help improve female health with a very important focus on the fact that we, as women, are not flawed or weak and that there are solutions to these struggles."

Katie – Wellness Mama, www.wellnessmama.com

"As you read *Lady Bits* you can feel Brianne's desire to inform and to educate women. Not only does she want you to understand and connect with your body, but she wants you to celebrate it. I couldn't help but be filled with this great pride to be a woman and to feel empowered to have such an amazing vessel carrying me through my ever-changing years!"

Tasha Mulligan MPT, ATC, CSCS
www.hab-it.com

"Right in line with my own work, Brianne talks about subjects that are typically considered taboo. She's not afraid to 'go there,' and yet she does so in a compassionate, friendly way that invites you to learn more. *Lady Bits* is a holistic and comprehensive approach to healthy living that's fun to read, perfect for women of all ages."

Nadya Andreeva, Author of Happy Belly
www.spinachandyoga.com

"*Lady Bits* is a gentle blend of yin and yang energy that exudes FEMININITY and HONORING oneself. Brianne is a genius when it comes to delivering information in a way that is not only impactful, but fun to read with a sprinkling of sexy – kind of like the author herself."

Jenn Edden, CHHC
www.jecoaching.com

LADY BITS

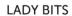

Lady Bits.

UNDERSTAND YOUR BODY,
ELEVATE YOUR HEALTH,
AND RECLAIM YOUR SPARK *naturally*

DR. BRIANNE GROGAN, DPT
Founder of FemFusion® Fitness

First Printing, 2015

Shine Press
www.femfusionfitness.com

Cover photo by Jessica Thompson
Cover design by Kelly Hampson
Edited by Libby Provost

ISBN 978-0692464519

IMPORTANT NOTE TO READERS:

*This book is for general informational purposes only. It contains the ideas and opinions of the author and is intended to provide helpful and informative material on the subjects addressed. It is not intended to diagnose or treat any medical condition(s) or to be used as a substitute for professional medical advice. **If you have, or think you have, a medical condition addressed in this book, please consult with a qualified healthcare practitioner.***

The author specifically disclaims all responsibility for any liability, loss, or risk, personal or otherwise, that is incurred as a consequence of the use and application of the contents of this book.

Any reference to or mention of manufacturers, products, or specific brands should not be interpreted as an endorsement or advertisement for any company or product.

The names and identifying information of some individuals referenced in this book have been changed. Any similarity to any person living or dead is merely coincidental.

Some of the material in this book has previously appeared under the author's name in the e-book FemFusion Fitness for Intimacy (© 2012), and online on the FemFusion Fitness website.

Visit www.femfusionfitness.com for information and encouragement related to women's health and wellness.

DEDICATION

*To my husband, who has tolerated my favorite form of entertainment –
thousands of hours of reading and listening to health and wellness books,
audiobooks, podcasts, and videos – and endured countless midnight
illuminations for me to scrawl notes and capture random musings for
this very book. Thank you for loving me for who I am. You are my best
friend, my rock, and my biggest fan. Without you, I would not have
had the opportunity to continue my FemFusion journey.
I love you more than words can express.*

*To my mom, a radiant example of healthy aging.
Thank you for being my first teacher, my first best friend, and my eternal
role model. I know we'll never discuss the parts of this book that make you
(and me!) blush, but I also know that you love and accept my creativity,
my passions, and the woman I've become.*

Table of Contents

PART III: REAL LIFE LESSONS IN RADIANT AGING

PART IV: THE PROPER CARE AND FEEDING OF A FEMALE BODY

PART V: LOVE YOUR BODY

PART VI: LOVE YOUR LOVE LIFE

Accept Changes
Surround Yourself With Romance
Harness the Power of Oxytocin
During Sex:
Mantra Magic
The Chakra Dance
Using Kegels to Enhance Intimacy
Kegels During Orgasm (Extra Credit Kegels)
Extending Orgasm
Position Considerations
Looking Ahead:
Keep it Spicy
Open Up and Lighten Up

PART VII: MAKING THE CHANGE

INTRODUCTION

Body shame is pervasive in society today. I have a friend who refers
to her yearly pelvic exam as her "annual humiliation," and I've known
several women who will only make love in the dark. We not only judge
ourselves (and others) by physical appearance, we also compare our
body's physiological functions and abilities to other women's and become
discouraged – as if we have somehow failed – when we don't measure
up or operate the way we think we should. We envy, we fret, we push,
and we try to morph and change, but until we understand and love
ourselves from the inside out, we will remain stuck, stagnant, or worse –
disillusioned and/or ill.

A glance at the cover and title of this book might lead you to the
conclusion that we are going to discuss sparking things up in the
bedroom, but that's only part of the story. *Lady Bits* is a comprehensive
resource to help you learn how to understand, care for, and love your
unique female body. *Lady Bits* is more than information – it's a complete
lifestyle program with tools that any woman can use in her own daily
life. The program culminates in a 14-Day Action Guide that incorporates
three steps for better sex, but first and foremost, *Lady Bits* informs and
empowers you to get intimate with your ultimate partner in life: YOU.

I want you to turn the final page knowing that radiant health isn't a
particular weight or size, or a certain look or style; rather, it's an attitude
and a way of living. Why? Because the more you get to know your body
and the better you take care of yourself, the more comfortable and secure
you'll be as a lover, mother, partner, and friend.

I have spent countless hours researching spirituality, fitness, nutrition,
and women's health, and now I'm thrilled to put the pieces together
for you. East meets west, strong pelvic floor meets sexy flat abs, chakra
balance meets hormonal balance, meditation meets sexual positions,
we're going to cover it all in a way that will leave you feeling energized
and excited, like you just had a great conversation with your best
girlfriend. My hope is that you'll laugh (and maybe even cry), nod your

head in agreement, and praise God that someone understands you.

Personally, I learn best through stories – when theory is brought to life through actual human experience. Throughout the following pages, I will share bits and pieces of my own health journey and introduce you to several of my friends and clients. I had the pleasure of conducting formal interviews with women of all ages while researching this book and have also been privy to questions, concerns, breakthroughs, and personal stories from clients in my health coaching practice and FemFusion group fitness classes. When you are done reading *Lady Bits*, I hope you not only feel more grounded and centered in yourself, but also that you have gained a whole new posse of female confidantes. ***Mostly, I want you to feel truly seen and to realize that whatever you're going through, you're normal.*** Whether it's PMS, pelvic pain, incontinence, or low libido, you're not "weird," and you're not alone.

Author Brené Brown is quoted as saying, "Shame cannot survive being spoken. It cannot survive empathy." I'm done with shame, aren't you? Body shame, fear of inadequacy, guilt related to imperfection... I've had enough. So let's chat.

"Question... Why 'Lady Bits?' Isn't that a tad crude?"

First, there's nothing crude about female genitalia, to which "lady bits" commonly refers. Prepare yourself: we will be discussing "lady bits" (in the most loving and respectful of ways)! But far beyond anatomy, I'm going to share "bits" of information that all women should know about their bodies, their health, and making the most of their personal wellness journeys. It's high time that women embrace and accept their bodies, and this begins with facts.

Knowledge is power.

We live in a fascinating time in which the worlds of health, fitness, and nutrition are experiencing a true renaissance. Old paradigms are being challenged, not just by scientists and researchers, but also by everyday people who are taking a critical look at the dogma we've accepted as true.

Something in modern Western society is not working. People are sicker, fatter, and unhappier than ever before, and LIFESTYLE appears to be one of the primary contributors to this epidemic of feeling "blah."

Although you might not have the time or interest to sort through the latest information on women's health and lifestyle, I have a bit of an obsession with it. Using my educational background and clinical knowledge as a doctor of physical therapy combined with dogged determination to expand my knowledge base by studying the experts, I have brought this information together for you.

WHO NEEDS TO READ *LADY BITS*, AND WHY

Lady Bits is intended for women of all ages, all over the world. Real women – just like you – who may not have medical training, but who know that there has to be a better, more natural way to get their spark back (to feel better, more energetic, and sexier) than the oft-prescribed combo of antidepressants, a restrictive low-fat diet, and punishing their bodies with fitness programs they don't enjoy.

I began my career as a women's health physical therapist. Over the past four years, I have not worked in a medical setting but have instead nurtured and grown my fitness and lifestyle business, FemFusion® Fitness. My current reality is heavily colored by the non-clinical "real life" experiences I've had working with women in my group exercise classes and health coaching interactions. I am no longer just speaking to women with diagnosed health conditions; rather, I'm speaking to "everywoman."

Let's call this "everywoman" Sally. Although no two women are exactly alike, take a peek...Sally might look a lot like YOU.

Sally is married and has two kids. She works full time and feels consumed by the pressures of work and family life. Balance? Yeah, right. There's no such thing! Sally is just getting by, forging ahead, and focusing her attention on the essentials. Between her kids' soccer and karate practices, weekly phone calls with her sister, being available to help her mother (who's caring for Sally's ailing grandma), monthly PTO meetings, and a standing commitment to her church group, Sally doesn't have time for herself. She's starting to lose touch with the things that make her "her."

Sally feels low energy and lethargic most of the time, and, honestly, she doesn't want to have sex anymore. She WANTS to want sex, but most of the time she's just too darn tired.

Losing the stubborn last ten pounds of baby weight (from baby number two, born seven years ago) has been hard for Sally. She can't eat like she used to be able to and then expect a week of dieting or a single gym session to take it off. Speaking of the gym, she's just not "into" those bootcamp classes her friends rave about. The last time she went, she hurt her back and she'd rather just play it safe.

Sally has been critical of her body since she was a teen. Her self-judgment has been made even worse by the weight gain and body changes from pregnancy and childbirth. **It kills her that she's said she hates her body in front of her children.** She knows that her kids are still young, but she also knows how quickly they pick up on these things. Sally is desperately concerned with her body image and negative self-talk and is ready to change that relationship...but she just doesn't know how to start.

Making the right food choices is another battle. Sally has constant sugar cravings and feels addicted to carbs. She needs coffee to get going in the morning and is regularly constipated or bloated...another reason she doesn't really "want it" (sex) the way she did when she was younger!

What does Sally really want? **To turn a few heads.** To feel light, confident, toned, graceful, and vibrant. For people to wonder, "What's her secret?" despite the fact that she's entering midlife and is starting to notice a few stray grays along with fine lines and wrinkles. Sally simply wants to FEEL BETTER. She knows that there's so much potential, but she doesn't know how to get there. She wants someone to give her a plan, because – honestly – she does better when someone tells her what to do. She needs someone to make it easy, and someone who understands her needs. She's willing to put in the effort – she has (a bit) more time now that both kids are in school – but she needs someone to lead the way.

Even if you don't identify with Sally – even if you're in college and can't fathom the idea of marriage and boredom in the bedroom, or if you're in your seventies and are reinventing yourself after retirement and possibly even a major life change such as divorce or widowhood – stick with me. You will benefit from the wisdom in this book. This wisdom does not come from me; rather, it comes THROUGH me from all of the wonderful teachers and mentors I have had over the years.

Throughout my research, tutelage, and personal experience, the primary lesson I've learned is this: **You have to see the dirt in order to clean the house.** So if you're really and truly ready for change, then *Lady Bits* is for you. Get to know your body and what to expect as you move through life, **bust through your blocks** when it comes to self-acceptance, self-love, and self-care, and then when you're ready, start the 14-Day Action Guide for a beautiful body and sizzling sex. If my system works for you, I guarantee you will want to stick with it for life.

As my friend and mentor Jessica Drummond (founder of the Integrative Pelvic Health Institute) says, "You can't hate your body into health. You have to LOVE your body into health."

Ladies, it's time to love yourself up. Let's get started.

PART I:
Sexy.
Confident.
Strong.

STOP EXISTING... START LIVING!

"The first wealth is health."
–Ralph Waldo Emerson

"The more I expand my inner awareness and spiritual faith,
the more conscious I am of how I feel. And as I grow more aware of
my physical well-being, it becomes harder to indulge in bad habits."
–Gabby Bernstein

"Go forth and set the world on fire."
–Ignatius of Loyola

Chapter 1

YOUR MOJO... WHERE DID IT GO?

You're standing in the doorway of your son's bedroom answering his relentless questions about quicksand and quasars. You don't know the answers, but you try to give reasonable, semi-educated responses that make you sound "adult" and knowledgeable. You extricate yourself by slowly backing away from his door as he pelts you with questions. Your answers become shorter and more clipped, and soon you're calling them out from the hallway as you retreat toward the envisioned solace of your bedroom. Nothing sounds better than slipping between the sheets and cracking the novel you haven't had a chance to read in weeks. But then you remember that there's another family member who needs you in an entirely different way: your husband. And you're exhausted.

Is this scene familiar to you?

We've all been there – fallen into bed at the end of a long day, wiped out, and suddenly realized, "I can't remember the last time I had sex!"

Sex is a significant part of most committed relationships. If we are to believe Hollywood, we should all be aching to jump between the sheets at a moment's notice no matter how fast life is moving. But the reality is that libido often takes a back seat to hectic schedules, shifting hormone levels, and fatigue from the many roles that women play (mother, grandmother, employee, employer, friend, partner, dog-walker, errand-runner, household organizer, and so on).

As a whole, women tend to be extremely disciplined. We multi-task, keep our families on track, and make plans and goals that we work diligently toward accomplishing. This discipline keeps our worlds turning, but there can be a cost: the freewheeling fun of romance and sexuality can be siphoned off to the end of our to-do lists. I know all about this; I am a list **master**, and I can say with a blend of pride and shame that until I learned to prioritize MYSELF, the tasks on my to-do list often trumped the downtime that is conducive – even necessary – for personal care and for nurturing my intimate life. This task-oriented approach to life allowed me to maintain a high level of fitness, keep a clean house, and accomplish big things professionally; however, it left my personal life lacking. Things changed when I added tasks related to self-care and intimacy to my daily to-do lists. It helped me reclaim my sexy, sparkly, glowing inner goddess, and I have a hunch it will work for you, too.

THE TRUE DEFINITION OF "SEXY"

What is sexy? Confidence! After spending the majority of my career promoting women's health, fitness, and "moving like a lady," I have determined that **confidence** is the number one quality that makes women feel desirable...and desire. We have all known confident women who simply radiate strength and sex appeal. They are magnificent. Irresistible!

Take a look at what the following women told me when I asked them, "What makes you feel sexy?" Every woman responded with her own individual spin on **confidence**.

Jessica, 34:
> *"My husband makes me feel sexy. The way he looks at me – like I'm the most beautiful thing he has ever seen. Even when I was nine months pregnant and feeling huge and uncomfortable in my own skin, one look from him made me feel confident and secure."*

Karen, 40:
> *"I feel sexy when I'm in charge. It makes me feel on top of my game, and that is sexy."*

Angela, 30:
> *"When it comes to feeling sexy, the biggest thing for me is feeling strong. I can tell a huge difference when I have been exercising regularly."*

Jess, 29:

> "I feel sexy when I wear nice clothes. I don't have to spend a lot of money to feel
> put together, I just need to take the time in the morning to dress myself well.
> Wearing a pretty sundress with leggings and a blazer instantly lifts my spirits
> and makes me feel confident. I can be just as comfy in leggings and a dress as I
> am in jeans and a sweatshirt, but I hold my head higher when I feel pretty."

What makes **you** feel confident?

At twenty, confidence may come from a great pair of jeans, killer heels, and the perfect lip-gloss. Granted, this may help in your thirties, but you will also get a boost from getting **back** into those jeans after baby, running your first road race, or jumping on a trampoline without needing to change your underwear. In your forties and fifties the surge of confidence may come when you are able to laugh with girlfriends over a few glasses of wine without a panty liner, when you can pull into the garage without having to sprint to the bathroom, or when you know you can still make your partner look twice when you walk through the room.

Overall, a huge aspect of confidence is **body confidence** – feeling comfortable and secure in your own skin. Body confidence means different things to different women, but in general, feeling fit, healthy, and in control of our bodies makes all of us feel secure and self-assured. Our health and bodily functions are things that most of us don't even think about...until we have to.

Check in with yourself: Do you feel confident today?
Do you have a strong sense of "body confidence?"

Are you in control of your bodily functions? No, really! Answer this question honestly. It's surprisingly common for slip-ups and mishaps to occur (i.e. bladder leakage), especially as you get older.

With confidence comes RADIANCE. Radiance is something that exudes from your entire being: your eyes, your smile, your aura. It's something that people sense and connect to on an entirely different level than that which can be seen (or even felt) in the physical realm.

You might think your external appearance is the first thing people notice when they meet you, but despite the temporary distraction of bright, shiny external appearances, most people – at least the interesting, intelligent, quality people you want to be around – aren't fooled by what they see on the outside. Rather, they feel your energy level and sense your overall "vibe." They see the way your eyes shine and the way you carry yourself, they hear your emotions and your mental health in your voice and in the words you choose.

Check in with yourself: What energy do you radiate?
How do you look at the world, and at yourself?
Are you willing to embrace new ideas and step outside your comfort zone?
Do you glow from the inside out?

When you stop feeling radiant, it shows. Poor lifestyle choices including overly processed foods, lack of exercise, and lack of self-love or feelings of low self-worth can dim your bright light. You begin to emit a negative energy that can be felt in yourself and by others around you.

Let's look a little deeper. What shakes your confidence? What dims your radiance?

Karen, 40:
  "My 'muffin top' – especially when I notice it during a workout!"

Mary, 62:
  "These days it's like, 'oh my God, I have to go [to the restroom] immediately!' I also leak a little when I laugh. In general, I feel like my muscle tone has really decreased as I have gotten older... everything sags – my neck, my breasts... There are folds everywhere."

Jess, 29:
  "Silly external things shake my confidence, like a pimple or a bad hair day. I have to remind myself that people are looking at my smile and listening to my words, they aren't focusing on my hair."

Jill, 37:
  "True story: I pulled on my favorite jeans and realized that I couldn't zip

Lady Bits

them up all the way. I felt physically ill, and very upset with myself. I couldn't think of a reason why this seemed to happen overnight, and now I had the added stress of rethinking my outfit, much less my diet. After I took them off I noticed a tear in the leg. How did that happen? On closer inspection I realized that they were not my jeans, they were my 14-year-old daughter's jeans, which are two sizes smaller than me, and what the heck? I almost fit into them! Talk about a mood swing. From depression to 'hot mama' in less than five minutes!"

For some women, weight gain or other issues related to appearance dim their inner light. For others, rushing through their workplace to make it to the restroom on time is a confidence shaker. And for other women, wondering, "where did my sex drive go?" and feeling that they "should" feel sensual (but don't) diminishes their radiance.

These issues can be difficult to control as we transition through our female life stages from pregnancy to postpartum, to menopause and beyond. The body changes. Hormones change. Strength changes. These changes are universal, and if you have experienced them, you are certainly not alone.

But what if I were to tell you that you could reclaim your sexy self – reclaim your confidence and RADIANCE – by understanding your body, accepting and appreciating yourself, and caring for yourself? What if I told you that you could prevent, treat, and even cure, issues such as incontinence and low libido using simple exercises coupled with a few easy lifestyle changes? You could save money, hassle, and embarrassment and feel sexier and empowered as you age. Would you make these changes? My hope – since you have picked up this book – is that you will say "yes!"

This is not just an exercise program, it is a **lifestyle program**. My motto is, "Eat clean, move every day, SHINE BRIGHTER." When you prioritize healthy living, you will stay fit, sexy, and confident for life, and you will reap more rewards than you can imagine.

Chapter 2

MY STORY

You're reading this book for a reason. Maybe your sex life has hit bottom. Maybe you want to lose a few pounds. I have a hunch you're not feeling terribly confident or radiant. Perhaps you are here because this time, you're actually ready for change?

If you're ready for change, I am ready to help. First, let me tell you a little bit about myself.

> **"Your mess is your message."**
> **–Author Unknown**

As previously mentioned, I am a doctor of physical therapy and the founder of FemFusion® Fitness. I refer to myself as a healthy "foodie," a fitness fanatic, and a passionate advocate for women's health.

Why do I care so much about women's health? It hearkens back to a message I saw emblazoned across a t-shirt one day. It said: ***If mama ain't happy, ain't nobody happy!*** I was a young girl at the time and I didn't understand the meaning, but for some reason, it stuck with me. Now, as a grown woman, I completely understand. **Happiness, feeling good, and taking care of your own health should be your primary focus as a woman in society today.** Does this sound hedonistic? It's not. Your health and happiness drives the health and happiness of your family and ultimately, the world at large.

I firmly believe that strong, healthy women are the backbone of a thriving society. Men may still make more money than women (on average), but women are the real influencers. Women talk, share, spread messages, and connect.

Despite the fact that many of us are employed outside of the home, women tend to be the primary caregivers and leaders within the family, making most of the decisions when it comes to lifestyle including scheduling activities, meal planning, and grocery shopping. We still do the lion's share of tending to and raising our children. **Thus, the way we live is the way the next generations will live.** This is why I share my "eat clean, move every day" message with women like you, globally: because women can change the health of the world.

This is your power, and your responsibility! **Making the world brighter starts and ends with YOU.** By sparking your own personal light, others around you will rise to your brilliance.

When I was working as a clinical physical therapist, I saw a huge need for prevention, and not just a secondary "cure" for disease or dysfunction that has already taken hold. I saw the benefits of healthy living, but also how frightening life can be when it goes by the wayside. From weight gain to back pain to premature aging...I saw it. And honestly, when I haven't taken my own health seriously, I've felt it. This is what makes my work so personal. Just like you, I have been on my own wellness journey with bumps, twists, turns, lots of highs, and plenty of lows. Thankfully, my vulnerabilities and weaknesses have become my strengths. Allow me to share my story.

MILESTONES AND TURNING POINTS

I wasn't always "into" fitness. As a child, I hated PE class, I was picked last for every team, and I was teased that I sprinted "like a chicken." But then I found long-distance running. I came to love the sensation of losing my thoughts as my feet drummed the pavement, over and over. I felt free...like I could fly. From that moment, I was hooked on the power of movement.

Time marched on. I completed my doctoral degree, got married, and became a mother. After my son was born, I was appalled to see saggy skin where a toned tummy had once been. I could not contract – or even sense – my abdominal muscles at all! I remember looking at my bare torso in the mirror and trying my hardest to flex my abdominals the way I could before pregnancy. Rather than see any type of muscular definition, I saw loose skin...lots of it.

Desperate to return to my former fit self I started running three weeks postpartum, long before my midwife cleared me to participate in such strenuous exercise. Needless to say, my body was not ready for the high impact of running. I paid for it with aching knees from ligaments that were still soft and loose from pregnancy, as well as disconcerting symptoms from a weak pelvic floor that was not ready to have my pelvic organs pounding into it, step after step. During my runs and even some of my longer walks, I noticed that I was leaking a small amount of urine. In addition, when I coughed I felt as though everything inside was "falling out." A feeling of heaviness in my pelvis and a look at my vagina with a handheld mirror confirmed what I feared: things had changed. I had mild pelvic organ prolapse from the strain I had placed on my weak, overstretched pelvic floor.

I had recently completed my initial coursework that allowed me to specialize in the field of women's health physical therapy, and yes, I should have known better than to run three weeks after childbirth! However, this mistake proved to be a blessing in disguise. I was able to learn from my experience and to empathize with patients who came to me with impairments related to pelvic floor weakness. I devoured books on the subject of core and pelvic floor health, and with this information combined with input from my colleagues, I came up with a fitness and lifestyle plan to treat my own symptoms. I followed my plan dutifully and after three months I was able to participate fully in my athletic endeavors without bladder leakage. Furthermore, the feeling of heaviness and "falling out" in my pelvic region resolved.

In January 2009 I began blogging about topics related to women's health and fitness. I had so much fun writing about women's issues, so much **passion** about women's health, and so much personal experience with fitness that I took a risk and decided to further develop a concept that had been evolving in my mind. In tandem with my work as a clinical physical therapist, I launched FemFusion® Fitness with the mission of helping women feel sexy, confident, and strong through movement. I began teaching group exercise classes in Portland, Oregon, as well as workshops that focused on inner core health and wellness.

But then, surprise! My husband was offered a job in Germany. Within two months we put our house on the market, packed up, and moved overseas. I decided to put FemFusion® Fitness on hold.

Initially, I was content being a stay-at-home mom. I didn't feel called to return to clinical physical therapy. But as we reached the six-month mark of our stint abroad I felt a burning desire to return to health and fitness. I deeply wanted to share my passion and knowledge with my new community. In fall 2011, I began teaching group exercise classes once again – this time in Germany – primarily to women involved in the US military community. I also wrote a book, titled *FemFusion Fitness for Intimacy*, which lives on as the "bones" of *Lady Bits*.

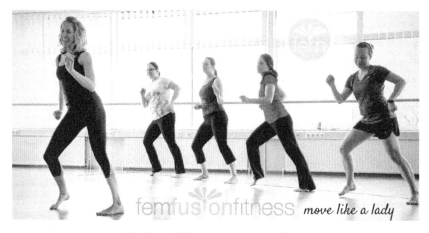

FemFusion® Fitness group exercise classes

I had always wanted to write for a larger audience, and by 2012, with my first book under my belt, I felt like I was on fire both personally and professionally. Always an over-achiever, I dove back into work, engulfing myself in busy-ness without taking even a moment to celebrate – or even consider – my recent accomplishments.

In addition to teaching my weekly group fitness classes, I also worked with multiple private fitness clients, picked up some physical therapy work in a local rehab clinic, completely revamped my website, created and produced 11 e-courses, took on the monumental task of learning how to navigate the worlds of online marketing and social media networking, began training to become a certified women's health and nutrition coach, created an online group health coaching program, continued blogging, and...oh yeah...tried to remain first and foremost a wife and mom with a semi-clean house cooking three meals from scratch each and every day.

Makes me tired just writing it.

By spring 2014 I felt broken, irritable, uninspired, exhausted, painful, antisocial, unsexy, and stuck. I had a painful itchy rash up and down my right leg, a buzzing in my chest, and a steel band of tension around my head. I felt like I was aging before my very eyes. Wrinkles set in fast and furiously, and I was not being my best self to my husband or my son. I had no motivation or inspiration for anything or anyone. I just wanted people to leave me alone! I knew something needed to change and I wasn't willing to seek assistance from medication. Instead I turned inward, DROPPED EVERYTHING, and took a break. I was stressed out, burned out, and deep down I knew that I needed rest, sleep, and relaxation. Not surprisingly, a tech-free family vacation and time off over the summer allowed me to reclaim my spark.

Summer 2014 was a healing time for me, but then fall rolled around. With my son back in school and a renewed zest for work and life, I jumped in – once again – to all of my personal and professional commitments. This time, my painful physical and emotional symptoms came back tenfold.

Two months in a row, I hit low points where I secretly – and seriously – researched ways to leave my husband and son. Not only did I want to be left alone, I wanted to leave everything. As you hear many clinically depressed (or even suicidal) people say, "I thought they'd be better off without me." Although I love my husband and son dearly and they had done nothing to harm me or push me away, I deeply and painfully wanted to either skip town, or skip out on life completely. These are some of the words I used to describe my feelings in my journal: debilitated, guilty, wrung out, crappy wife, and terrible mom.

My husband, who knew I'd hit bottom, finally nudged (okay, dragged) me to a psychotherapist. After just a few sessions I started to feel better. I gained clarity about what I wanted in my business and my life. My dreams changed from recurring nightmares of getting lost in huge spooky houses and mazes of dark, dusty rooms, to thrilling adventures and exciting treasure hunts. I started to know, understand, and appreciate myself. My mood lightened. My family was happier. I was so much happier!

But then BOOM – it hit again. I felt just as low as I did when I started therapy a month prior, and I was so let down. Luckily, my mental capacities were strong enough to allow me to take a critical look at the calendar and use my professional training in women's health to make some connections. I realized that the day I called my therapist to schedule my first appointment was exactly four weeks (28 days) prior. As you probably know, the average menstrual cycle is 28 days. When I started tracking my moods along with my cycle I noticed a trend that had been increasing over the past year.

For the first time in my life, in my mid-thirties, PMS struck, and it struck hard.

This is not to say that therapy wasn't helpful (or necessary) for me... It was, but it wasn't the end of the line. It was just another healing modality to help support and piece together the unique puzzle of "me." From learning how to properly manage diet and exercise, stress levels, heal my emotional burdens and self-worth issues, clarify my passion and purpose, and navigate the delicate dance of hormones, I had a lot to figure out in order to reclaim my radiance.

Through this rollercoaster ride I learned the following important lesson: people – particularly women – are more sensitive than they might think (or be willing to admit).

How about you? Do you notice changes in your mood, energy level, or sleep patterns when the seasons change? Or when there's a full moon? As you age? With your menstrual cycle? If so, you're not alone, and you're not making it up.

You are not flawed.
You are not weak.
You are a woman!

You may change over time (in fact, I can guarantee you will), so you need to learn about your amazing female body and physiology in order to understand yourself, accept yourself, LOVE yourself, and be the radiant, sexy being you were born to be.

"But OTHER women (insert feared fatal flaw here)..."

"Other women don't make a big deal about it... Other women have amazing, hot sex every day... Other women can work 60 hours a week and feel fine... Other women get by on four hours of sleep per night... Other women can eat anything they want without gaining weight or developing food sensitivities... Other women experience menstrual cycles or menopause without going insane..."

Well guess what – you're NOT other women. You are your own unique person and you are not imagining it if you have issues that other women don't (appear to) have. It's okay!

I identify as a highly sensitive individual, and if you're reading this, my guess is that you do too. If you were drawn to my tagline of "move like a lady," or if you purchased this book because you're interested in deepening your relationship with not only your partner but also YOURSELF, then you are an intuitive, sensitive being as well.

We are all just bodies of energy having a human experience. There is energy all around us, and certainly within us, and we can't help but absorb EVERYTHING at some level. It's no wonder that we (as a culture) are stressed out, strung out, and feeling less-than-radiant. It's no wonder that I was. Thankfully, I found a way to reclaim my spark.

That's why I'm here with you right now – to spread the message that the radiance and sexiness that you desire is an INSIDE job, and it's attainable through simple and natural lifestyle modifications and a little bit of education.

Today, a hearteningly rapid six months after my fall 2014 "crash," I've hit that sweet spot of LOVING movement, eating healthfully, doing my best to stress less and sleep more, and overall, just trying to enjoy the ride. Ultimately, these are the keys to health, and my mission is to help YOU feel the same. Energetic. Vibrant. Sexy. Fit. Strong. Sounds good, doesn't it?

Enough about me. Let's talk about the subject of this book...YOU!

Chapter 3

THE VALUE OF INNER CORE WELLNESS

Many women are uncomfortable talking about the inner core (which includes the pelvic floor), as well as the inevitable use of the word "vagina." I have heard women call their vaginas any and all of the following: vajayjay, nether-regions, hoo-haw, lady-parts, girlie-bits, undercarriage, and simply "down there." Many women who do not have issues related to their pelvic floor muscles look at me with blank expressions when I describe what I do for a living, and when I explain the importance of preventive pelvic floor health and wellness. They do not understand the implications of inner core weakness, or the problems that can arise when the pelvic floor isn't properly protected throughout life. I cringe when this happens, because I know that as time marches on, most of them will come to understand the implications firsthand.

My journey has been buoyed by talking with hundreds of females inside and outside of the clinical (physical therapy) and fitness settings. I have heard countless women say, "I had no idea that there was treatment for this kind of problem," referring to incontinence, prolapse, pain with intercourse, low libido, etc., and, "My friends have the same problems. I'll have to tell them that there's help!" After receiving this type of feedback time and again, I realized how common these issues are and how many women could benefit from some basic knowledge about inner core health, as well as their amazing bodies in general. I became inspired to write **this book** with the goal of creating a holistic lifestyle and fitness program that addresses women's needs when it comes to radiance of the mind, body, and spirit. Most importantly, I wanted the information to be fun, accessible, easy to learn, and comfortable. In short, I wanted to take the "ick" factor out of discussing the pelvic floor, continence, sexual health, and other "lady bits."

"I'm confused. Why are these 'inside' (inner core) muscles so important?"

When the inner core is strong and working well, pelvic organs are held in place, you don't leak when you sneeze, intercourse is stimulating and pain free, your back does not hurt, and balance is not a concern. When the inner core is overly clenched or extremely weak and lax, particularly the pelvic floor (for example, after childbirth or pelvic trauma, or with deconditioning that results from a sedentary lifestyle), the following problems can occur:

- Back and/or pelvic pain
- Difficulty with arousal and/or vaginal lubrication
- Bladder, uterine, or rectal prolapse
- Incontinence
- Instability of the trunk and pelvis, contributing to balance problems (ultimately increasing your risk of falls and fractures)

As a woman, you will likely encounter at least one of these issues at some point. Thus, strengthening and maintaining the muscles of the inner core is vitally important to your body – and to your life – as a whole.

The purpose of *Lady Bits* is not only to spice things up in the bedroom, but also to educate you about your female anatomy, help you connect with your inner core, and to provide strategies for a lifetime of wellness. If you feel that you are not ready for the information ahead or if you feel that you have an impairment that is unfit for (or unresponsive to) this program, please speak to your doctor or refer to the Resources section at the end of the book. I want everyone to reach the final page feeling satisfied that they have the information they need to independently continue their own personal journey toward improved inner core fitness and enhanced intimacy.

THE IMPORTANCE OF SELF-CARE

"You, yourself, as much as anybody in the entire universe, deserve your love and affection."
–Buddha

As stated in Chapter 2, I truly believe that strong, happy women are the backbone of a strong, happy society. By doing yourself a favor and taking care of yourself, you're actually doing the WORLD a favor. For the helpful, compassionate, caring and service-minded woman that I know you are, this should help justify the need to take some extra time and effort on behalf of yourself!

Like flight attendants tell you when flying: "Put on your oxygen mask first before assisting others." You must serve yourself so that you can best "show up" for everyone else. If you don't, all you're going to show – or give – is resentment.

You may not realize how many people you influence; make sure that your (sometimes unintended) influence is positive. Eat clean, move every day, get plenty of sleep, take time for yourself, and foster healthy relationships. You will be happier, those around you will be happier and better cared for, and – ultimately – this is how you can make the world a better place.

Self-care is quite a journey and one that many women "forget" to take due to the pressures of daily life, family, work, etc. I am thrilled to see that you're interested in listening to your body, respecting your needs, and treating yourself well, because you are your own best friend. No one can take care of yourself better than YOU can.

I began my personal development journey many years ago, and ultimately learned that it wasn't about getting "somewhere," or getting "better" so that I could do or become a certain "thing" or look a certain way. It wasn't a step-wise process with a specific end point. Rather, it was a path of inner work with the ultimate goals being self-acceptance, self-love, and seeing (and valuing) my own worth. Without that, I couldn't achieve anything else. Loving myself and learning how to properly care for myself was actually the "secret" that allowed everything else to fall into place.

Please take this seriously. It will work for you, too.

Chapter 4

HOW TO USE THIS BOOK

"Let's get down to business. Core fitness and self-care can lead to a beautiful body and better sex?"

ABSOLUTELY! This book is going to show you why (and how).

This is not a passive book – it's an active book! As you read I encourage you to take notes, take pauses to ask yourself questions and try out the exercises, and of course there are the digital workouts and the 14-Day Action Guide for you to explore.

Books that are solely informational aren't practical enough for me. I like a plan. But on the flip side, I often feel like a failure after reading books that are 100% action-oriented, because I can't seem to stick to the plan if it's not backed by a solid foundation or reason "why." That's why I wrote this book as a gradual progression for the reader.

First, you will build a strong base of knowledge about your body (anatomy, physiology, and changes that may take place throughout your life).

Building upon that strong foundation, you will learn how to properly care for yourself. Think of this as your toolbox for better health, including fitness, nutrition, self-care, and self-love techniques, as well as specific action items, such as my fun and effective Inner Core Energizer routine.

Finally – really honing in – you will apply everything you've learned to the *Lady Bits* three-step system for sizzling sex.

The 14-Day Action Guide at the conclusion of *Lady Bits* is intended for readers who are less "do it yourself" and more interested in following a done-for-you plan.

There are many different types of readers. Some will pore over every page, completing each instruction step-by-step. Others will zip through the book, look at the pictures, and pick and choose the information they want to use. Knowing that this spectrum exists, I am going to highlight specific sections that I encourage every reader to truly focus on, even those who just flip through the program. Although each section in this book is an important part of the *Lady Bits* program, the selected items below are essential for learning more about your female anatomy, increasing body awareness, and improving circulation and muscular activation in the pelvic region.

If you want to get the most out of this program, read everything. If you are a "flipper," please hone in on the following sections:

- We Have to Talk About This (Chapter 5)
- Come on, Take a Look! (Chapter 7)
- Core Breathing (Chapter 11)
- Inner Core Energizer (Chapter 13)
- 14-Day Action Guide (Chapter 24)

Again, you will get the most out of this book if you read it thoroughly, without skipping a section. Take your time moving through the chapters. Do not rush; really "digest" each chapter. Your health, your body confidence – and ultimately, your sex life – will be the better for it.

GLOSSARY

The following is a list of definitions for terms you will see regularly throughout this book. Mark this section; you may need to return to it for reference.

Abductor (muscles) and Abduction: Abduction refers to movement of a body part away from the midline of the body. In the context of this book, I primarily refer to hip "abductors," also known as your outer hip and thigh muscles.

Adductor (muscles) and Adduction: Adduction refers to movement of a body part toward the midline of the body. In the context of this book, I primarily refer to hip "adductors," also known as your inner thigh muscles.

Biofeedback: Biofeedback typically refers to electronic monitoring of certain bodily functions (for example, heart rate or muscular control) in order to train patients to acquire voluntary control of that function. In the context of this book, I primarily use the term "biofeedback" to describe self-monitoring (via sight and/or physical touch) to help you improve voluntary control of your pelvic floor muscles.

Breathing Diaphragm, or Diaphragm: The dome-shaped muscle that separates the thoracic cavity (which contains the lungs) from the abdominal cavity. The diaphragm moves downward as you inhale (breathe in) and upward as you exhale (breathe out).

Core: A general term that refers to the deep and superficial muscles that stabilize, align, and move the trunk of the body. Also known as the "powerhouse" of the body.

Extensor (muscles) and Extension: Extension is the movement by which the ends of any jointed part are drawn away from each other, or "straightened." Extension allows the angle between the jointed bones to increase. In the context of this book, I primarily refer to hip "extensors," also known as your gluteal (glute) or butt muscles. I also refer to trunk extensors, indicating your back muscles.

Flexor (muscles) and Flexion: Flexion is a bending movement that decreases the angle between the bones at a joint. In the context of this book, I primarily refer to hip "flexors," such as your iliopsoas muscles. I also refer to trunk flexors, indicating certain abdominal muscles.

Hormone: A chemical messenger that circulates throughout your body and produces a specific effect, usually at a point remote from its origin. For example, the adrenal glands (which sit just above your kidneys) send out stress hormones, such as cortisol, that act on your brain, heart, metabolism, immune system, and more.

Inner Core: The deep muscles of the core and the focus of this book. The inner core muscles include the pelvic floor, the deep abdominals (transversus abdominis and internal and external obliques), the deep back muscles (erector spinae and multifidus), and the breathing diaphragm.

Intra-Abdominal Pressure: A term referring to the degree of pressure within the abdominal cavity. The abdominal cavity is bounded by the diaphragm (above) and the pelvic cavity (below).

Kegel(s): The term used to describe pelvic floor muscle exercises. This exercise was named after Dr. Arnold Kegel, M.D., F.A.C.S. (1894–1981).

Neutral Spine: A position in which the spine and pelvis are kept in ideal alignment, maintaining the natural curves of the spine.

Pelvic Brace: The act of contracting the pelvic floor muscles prior to an increase in intra-abdominal pressure. You can think of a pelvic brace as "sealing off" the openings in the pelvic floor.

Pelvic Floor: A group of muscles at the base of the pelvis that support the pelvic organs and help close off the urethra to stop the flow of urine. You may have heard these muscles be called PC muscles (named for the pubococcygeus, one of the muscles that make up the pelvic floor), kegel muscles, or even "love muscles."

Prolapse: A condition in which one or more of the pelvic organs (uterus, bladder, or rectum) shift out of their normal positions and press downward into the vaginal wall. The intestines can also prolapse, as well as the vaginal vault (top of the vagina) in women who have had a hysterectomy (surgical removal of the uterus).

Urinary Incontinence: Unintentional leakage of urine – even a small amount. Urinary incontinence can be further divided into subcategories of urge incontinence (leakage with a strong urge to urinate), stress incontinence (leakage during a physical activity or when involuntary pressure is put on the bladder, such as during a cough, sneeze, lift, or laugh), or mixed incontinence (a combination of urge and stress incontinence).

PART II:
Understand your Body

TO KNOW YOURSELF IS
TO LOVE YOURSELF.

"We must claim our bodies as our own to love and honor in their infinite shapes and sizes. Fat, thin, soft, hard, puckered, smooth, our bodies are our homes."
–Abra Fortune

"It is the absence of facts that frightens people: The gap you open, into which they pour their fears, fantasies, desires."
–Hilary Mantel

"Any fool can know. The point is to understand."
–Albert Einstein

Chapter 5

GETTING TO KNOW YOU

"Half of 26 to 35-year-olds couldn't identify a vagina on a picture of the female reproductive system, survey found."
–DailyMail UK[1]

WE HAVE TO TALK ABOUT THIS

I've said it to my clients and I'll say it now, to you... **You have a right – and a responsibility – to know your body better than your partner does.**

As quoted above, a study by women's cancer charity The Eve Appeal found that half of 26- to 35-year-olds couldn't identify the vagina on a diagram of the female reproductive system.[1] This is disturbing, since 26- to 35-year-old women are in their prime childbearing years...a time when women should absolutely know and understand their own reproductive anatomy! Study participants were asked to identify the vagina on a cross-sectional diagram of the uterus and vaginal canal. Many women think of the vagina as the "opening" or the "hole" and not the entire canal, which might have contributed to the confusion. But confusing or not, this study illustrates that **basic anatomical education is lacking amongst women.** One of my missions in life is to help women get to know their bodies and clear up any misinformation – or shame – surrounding them. Unfortunately, genital ignorance is experienced by many women in society today.

So let's get it all out there and talk details. Let's talk about your lady bits.

LADY BITS

Your vagina is more than just a "hole." Rather, the vagina consists of the canal between the cervix (the base of the uterus) and the external opening from which babies and menstrual blood can exit, and into which a penis or tampon can enter. In short, the vagina includes the canal and the "hole!"

The labia are the "lips" that help to enclose and protect the clitoris and the openings of the vagina and the urethra. The labia majora are the outermost lips and the labia minora are the innermost. In some women, the labia minora are completely hidden inside the labia majora and not visible externally. In other women, the labia minora protrude. **Both scenarios are completely normal!** Unfortunately, due in large part to body comparison and idealization made possible by the pornography industry, some women feel ashamed of their natural – and completely healthy – variations, and are turning toward labiaplasty (plastic surgery to change the appearance of the labia). This trend – dubbed "designer vagina" – is growing at an alarming rate, increasing five-fold between 2001 and 2010.[2]

Anterior to the vagina (more toward the front of your body) is the opening of the urethra. The urethra is the "tube" that leads from the bladder to the vulvar vestibule (the area inside the inner lips of the vulva where the vagina is found). The urethra conveys urine. In males, the urethra is much longer, and also conveys semen.

Anterior to the urethra (even closer to the front of your body) is the clitoris, an exquisitely sensitive area with one job: sexual pleasure. Interestingly, the clitoris is actually quite large! When you visualize the clitoris, think of a wishbone. The visible "button-like" portion that can be seen anterior to the urethra is just a small part of the entire structure. Clitoral tissue extends toward the pubic bone, is found in the anterior vaginal wall, and has "legs" of nerve endings that run along either side of the vaginal opening.

When you hear the word "vulva," the classic *Seinfeld* episode where Jerry mistakenly calls his date "Mulva" might come to mind faster than the actual definition (or location) of the vulva. If you don't know what – or where – your vulva is, you're not alone. The vaginal opening, the labia (both sets), the urethral opening, and the clitoris are all part of the vulva.

Essentially, the vulva is all of the external parts of your "private area."

The external portions of the vulva are hair-covered. Despite a rising trend that would have you believe otherwise, pubic hair is natural and totally okay. It does not need to be trimmed, shaved, waxed, or otherwise modified or removed unless you have a personal preference to do so. Relax and save some money and time. Cancel your next depilatory session!

The perineum, not technically a part of the vulva, is the area between your vagina and anus. This region is commonly referred to as the "taint" (slang). Episiotomies (surgical incisions intended to facilitate childbirth – a medical practice of debatable value) are completed in the perineum.

The anus is the end of the digestive tract, the opening from which feces exit the body.

We could get much more technical and detailed, but the above information covers the "basics" when it comes to your external genitalia. A few key points to remember: Your vulva is your entire "private area." Your vagina is more than just the "hole." The vagina connects the outer world to your inner world. Speaking of your inner world, let's go deeper.

WOMB POWER

The uterus – otherwise known as your womb – is a muscular organ that lies in your pelvic cavity between your bladder and rectum. The uterus is composed of the fundus (the dome shaped portion at the top), the body (the largest tapering central portion) and the cervix (which opens into the vagina). Pound for pound, the myometrial layer of the uterus is the strongest muscle in the female body.

Energetically, the uterus plays a very special role. It is our center of creativity and intuition – the very place from which all life begins. In women who bear children, the uterus houses and nurtures the developing baby, and its strong, muscular contractions help deliver the baby into the world. For women who do not bear children, the womb remains a center of pure creative potential: from business endeavors to art and relationships, anything that requires creative energy can be (energetically) "birthed" from – and felt in – the center, or root, of your body.

"Is there any scientific evidence for this? Where's the proof?"

The proof is in your body.

I have written this book to be as evidence-based as possible, drawing upon information gleaned from my post-graduate studies as well as current research. Information about womb energy is not found in peer-reviewed scientific journals, but I would be remiss if I did not share the vital role your prana – the life-force energy that flows in currents in and around your body – plays in your health. Information about prana has been passed down through the ages, and continues to be noted and observed in individual case studies and clinical examples amongst practitioners of energy medicine. Although I am not a trained practitioner of energy medicine, I have had several personal experiences with sensing – and shifting – the energy in my own body. My experiences, coupled with reports from women I've worked with and known, has convinced me that there is substance to the theory of womb energy specifically, and prana in general.

Scientific evidence is inarguably valuable, but it's not everything. Did our ancestors conduct formal research studies? No. They recognized what worked and what didn't, and they focused on continuing with, and building upon, the former. They passed down this information from generation to generation. They may not have known exactly why or how things worked, and they may not have had calculated 95% confidence intervals or other indicates of statistical significance, but that doesn't make their time-tested insights any less important or valid.

Throughout history and crossing cultural boundaries, generations of people – healers and grandmothers and "regular Joes" alike – understood the value of keeping a healthy stream of energy flowing throughout their bodies. For women, the uterus was, and still is, the center of this pranic flow.

Check in with yourself: Does this seem a little woo-woo to you? A little "out there?" Regardless, I encourage you to try the following exercise.

> ### EXERCISE – Womb Power:
>
> *Place your hands over your womb. Let your mind clear and your body relax. Open yourself to the idea of energy flowing through your body. What do you feel when you place your hands (physically) and your attention (mentally, spiritually, and energetically) over your womb? Take a moment to consider this, and then continue reading.*

Your uterus – which is seated within your pelvic bowl – is your creative center, your power center, your primal, energetically charged, sacred feminine center. Holistic women's healthcare provider and author Tami Kent states in her book *Wild Creative*, "This creative [energy] field exists not just in the pelvic bowl but around the whole body. It reflects the imprints and intelligence of the pelvic bowl, however, because this is where our body and energy are first created."[3]

It really is amazing to think that we, as women, developed and came into being within and through our mother's uterus. Even in utero, we had tiny, developing wombs of our own. We were nourished in this field of pure creative potential, and ultimately birthed with the ability to bear new life from our own womb in the future.

Is this too heady for you? Try to stay open and keep going with this exercise. It can be life changing.

Let's get back to the exercise. Return your attention to your womb. Again consider: What do you feel?

You might feel warmth or a sense of energetic "presence" in your womb. You might feel a sense of engorgement depending on where you are in your menstrual cycle, or even a pulsing or buzzing sensation; however, you may also feel nothing. You might feel coldness or emptiness, indicating stress or a lack of connection to your feminine center. This is not uncommon today in our fast-paced, male-dominated culture. Kent states that in her private healthcare practice, one of the common imbalances she sees is an **overactive masculine energy flow with an absent or diminished feminine energy flow**.[3] This is attributed to our culture's general emphasis on production, achievement, and building a career outside of the home, which at one time applied primarily to men and now applies to women as well.

If you feel a sense of coldness, emptiness, dullness, or stagnation (rather than warm, lively, freely flowing energy), then I suggest the following. First, tune into the "big picture" of energy moving throughout your body. Begin with the familiar visualization of blood circulating throughout your vessels, from your big arteries and veins to the tiny little capillaries in your fingertips and toes. Your circulatory system touches every nook and cranny of your internal body. Now shift your focus to your energetic system. Just as the circulatory system moves throughout your entire body, filling all of the internal spaces, so too does your energetic system. Feel your prana circulating throughout your body, and then bring awareness to your womb. What are you feeling now?

Kent states, "Women tend to fuel their energy with sheer willpower rather than from feminine inspiration, often depleting their essence, happiness, libido, and so on."[3] To counter this tendency, tune in to the energy flowing throughout your body with a special focus on the womb region. When you begin to connect with this feminine energy, you will notice a subtle – but powerful – shift that causes you to feel more centered and relaxed.

I suggest you return to this exercise on a regular basis as you move through this book. What may start as *"What the heck is she talking about?"* just might evolve into a profound relationship with your energetic female center. Personally, I like to place my hands over my uterus every night before I fall asleep. I take a few minutes to tune in to the flow of pranic energy coursing through my energetic center (or not, depending on my current mood or state of being). If I feel a cold or numb sensation over my womb, I gently focus my attention on it until the energy begins flowing. This simple practice calms me, grounds me, and brings me back to the power – and creative potential – that is my birthright.

THE MENSTRUAL CYCLE

Shame, fear, mistrust, indifference, and annoyance can all be used to describe women's feelings toward their bodies and bodily functions. For many of us, menstruation is (or has become) a source of embarrassment and hassle. We hide our tampons underneath other purchases and avoid eye contact with our checker or bagger. We use "sanitary products" to keep "clean and fresh," and we roll our eyes with shared understanding as we commiserate about our "time of the month." These murmured comments are often cloaked in mystery to the men and children in our lives; in fact, many women never refer to their "female issues" by proper names, anatomy, or purpose.

It doesn't have to be this way.

If you're still menstruating, your cycle is important to embrace and understand, at least at a basic level. Let's face it; unless you utilize Natural Family Planning or the Fertility Awareness Method of contraception, you probably do NOT understand menstruation. I didn't until recently, and my career is based on women's health and wellness!

The menstrual cycle is regulated by your sex hormones, which produce changes in the reproductive organs every 28 days (or so). Although an average cycle is 28 days, a healthy menstrual cycle can vary a few days in either direction with no ill effects. If your cycle is shorter than 21 days or longer than 35, consult with a healthcare professional who can help you troubleshoot. It is likely that some type of hormonal imbalance – which may be related to perimenopause and/or extreme stress, inflammation, poor gut health, or other significant issue(s) – is at the root.

The menstrual cycle is counted from the beginning of one menstrual period to the beginning of the next, and it is divided into three distinct phases: the follicular, ovulation, and the luteal phases. I will describe these phases in brief (they're quite complex), and will also correlate typical mood and productivity changes that you may note throughout your own cycle. It's a fascinating, beautiful ebb and flow that every woman should know.

The key to menstrual peace is learning how to flow with, and be open to, the changes in your energy, creativity, and mood throughout your cycle. Even when writing this book it was very clear to me that there were days when the words just flew onto the page, and others when I absolutely did not feel like writing AT ALL. Because I track my cycle so closely I was able to prepare for these shifts and not berate myself for being "lazy" or unproductive.

I encourage you to study this information and begin tracking your own cycle. Even if you're not tracking your cycle for fertility or family planning, it's interesting, enlightening, and may help you make some connections. And if you have a daughter, please share this information with her. Be the light... Show her how magical her body truly is!

> **Fun Tidbit:** Technology meets Fertility... "There's an app for that!" If you have a smartphone, a convenient way to keep track of your menstrual cycle is with an application such as "Period Tracker" (at the time of this writing, the "Lite" version is free). Period Tracker calculates the average length of your last three cycles, so it can more accurately predict the date your flow is going to show up. It also allows you to add notes about your symptoms so you can track your physical and emotional changes throughout the month.
>
> Interested in conception? A cervical ring called "Bloom" (newly introduced to the marketplace by Prima-Temp) wirelessly transmits your core body temperature to an app, continuously monitoring and detecting elevations in your base body temperature, a prime indicator of ovulation. As stated on their website, www.bloomring.com, it "pinpoints the window of fertility, without having to actively engage in data collection." No more thermometers... Now you can just glance at your cell phone!

Follicular Phase (days 1-13, on average)

Menstruation (when you begin bleeding, or "start your period") marks the beginning of the follicular phase. This is considered day one of your cycle, when your body realizes that you are not, in fact, pregnant, and the innermost lining of the uterus begins to break down and shed.

On day 1 (the first day of your period), hormone levels have plummeted and estrogen and progesterone are the lowest they will be throughout the cycle. These low levels of estrogen and progesterone signal the pituitary gland to produce Follicle Stimulating Hormone (FSH). FSH triggers small follicles – structures in the ovaries that support and grow your eggs – to mature. Your body is gearing up to "try again" next month!

The follicles and the eggs within produce estrogen in order to prepare the uterus for pregnancy. Often referred to as the "growing" or "building" hormone, estrogen is responsible for growing and maturing the uterine lining, and it also matures the egg prior to ovulation.

> **Fun Tidbit:** A female baby is born with all the eggs that she will ever have, estimated to be around two million. By the time she reaches puberty, this number has decreased to about 400,000. From puberty to menopause, only about 400-500 eggs will reach maturity and be released from the ovary (ovulation), rendering them capable of fertilization.[4]

Throughout the follicular phase, estrogen rises, and with it, your mood may elevate as well. By days 3-5 of the follicular phase you may begin feeling more confident and powerful. By days 6-7 your period should be completely or almost gone. By days 9-13 estrogen is at its peak, and you may be feeling particularly creative and confident.[5] In fact, the week preceding ovulation is often referred to as your "Venus Week," named after the Roman goddess of love, sex, beauty, and fertility.[6] During "Venus Week" all of your hormones are balanced in such a way that you may feel more energetic and charismatic, and for many women, more sexual. In other women, the charisma manifests less as sexual desire but more as creative energy. All of this charisma tends to peak just before ovulation, which marks the end of the follicular phase.

It is important to note that the length of the follicular phase is variable and can be affected by diet, stress, or illness. Thus, it can be tricky to predict your exact day of ovulation. If you are using Natural Family Planning or the Fertility Awareness Method of contraception, you will need to research the signs of ovulation to best promote or prevent pregnancy.

Ovulation (day 14, on average)

Today is a game-changer: the day that a sudden spike in Luteinizing Hormone (LH) causes a fully mature egg to burst through the wall of one of your ovaries. Most women alternate which ovary will produce an egg each month.

The egg moves through that ovary's fallopian tube, and then enters the uterus. Some women literally feel ovulation and experience "mittelschmerz" (yes, that's a real term meaning "middle pain" in German), which can cause slight pain or discomfort in the ovulating ovary.

Around ovulation, you might notice some slippery, clear mucous when you wipe after using the toilet. This is cervical mucus (looks and feels like egg whites), which helps move the sperm toward the egg and protects sperm from the acidity of the vagina.

If you are trying to conceive, now (and the 2-3 days leading up to now) is the time! But if you want to prevent pregnancy and are not using any other form of birth control, you will need to be extremely careful around ovulation time. **Sperm can live as long as 7 days inside the female body, so you will need to practice prophylaxis (i.e. condom use) during the entire week before ovulation.** After ovulation, the egg can live up to 24 hours without being fertilized, so you will need to practice prophylaxis for at least two days after you ovulate.

Luteal Phase (days 15-28, on average)

The remains of the follicle (the structure in the ovary that housed the egg) is called the corpus luteum. The corpus luteum produces large amounts of progesterone, which is known as the "pregnancy hormone" or the "relaxing hormone." Progesterone's main job is to help mature and maintain the uterine lining. Basically, it's padding things up to make the uterus as comfortable and snug as possible in case the egg is fertilized and there is a pregnancy.

Progesterone dominates during the luteal phase, and estrogen and testosterone levels are fairly low, especially during the first part of the luteal phase (around days 17-18). This can leave you feeling low-energy and possibly vulnerable. It's a good time for a quiet movie night with your friends, but probably not the best time to run a marathon or plan a hot date.

In the middle of the luteal phase (around days 21-24), progesterone is at its highest, and estrogen surges just a bit. Due to progesterone's bonding influence and estrogen's powerful creative, energetic, and "building" influence, this is a great time to tap into your intuition and work on relationship-building or creative projects with harmony and flow. Your nighttime dreams might be particularly colorful during your luteal phase.

Keep in mind, however, that symptoms of premenstrual syndrome (PMS) tend to begin around days 23-25 and may not wind down until days 27-28. **This is NOT the time to get on the scale.** Premenstrual fluid retention is a real thing...and so are the mood swings that can accompany PMS. Be extra kind to yourself during this time.

If the egg is NOT fertilized and conception or implantation does not occur, the corpus luteum will shrivel about 14 days after ovulation (day 28). This causes a sharp decrease in both estrogen and progesterone, triggering the onset of menstruation...and the cycle begins again. Self-care is at the top of your to-do list right now. Go book that mani-pedi and massage!

> **Fun Tidbit:** *Did you know that the moon and women's menstrual cycles are thought to be linked?* While there is not peer-reviewed, double-blinded, placebo-controlled scientific evidence to prove this phenomenon, the theory has stood the test

of time and is something worth exploring. Let's look a little closer, with the help of Elle Griffin, an expert in fertility and spirituality and the founder of *Over the Moon Magazine*.

According to Griffin, things are changing due to the introduction of hormonal birth control, artificial light, and the ability to be awake and productive around-the-clock, but traditionally, the female cycle has been connected to the fullness of the moon. The full moon has long been known as a peak time for fertility, not just for farmers and seed-planting, but also for baby-making. As Griffin writes:

"You've heard that the moon is what causes the tides. That beautiful force of gravity that operates between the sun, the moon, and the rotation of the earth results in a cosmic lunar pull on bodies of water and even, well, your bodies! The moon makes a complete orbit around the earth every 28 days (well 27.3 but who's counting). Similarly a woman's (regulated) menstrual cycle is 28 days in length. Coincidence?? Not at all!"[7]

When the sun, Earth, and the moon form a line, we see a "full moon," or a "new moon." In both cases, this alignment creates exceptionally strong gravitational forces on the earth and a pull, not only on the tides, but also within our bodies. **Thus, both the full moon and the new moon are times of release.**

Griffin states that modern women are divided into three groups. The first (and largest) group ovulates with the full moon and bleeds with the new moon. This is the most traditional group, mirroring our ancestors who planned weddings just prior to the full moon in order to provide the best chance for conception. Interestingly, our female ancestors most likely cycled as a group due to the phenomenon of menstrual synchronization (when women living in close proximity menstruate together), coupled with in-sync circadian rhythms. Since everyone lived naturally, by the light of the sun and the moon, the entire community would have tracked the cycles of the moon and noted its cyclical effect on their bodies and their lives.

The second group – a group that is growing as women's societal roles shift and change – ovulates with the new moon and bleeds with the full moon. These women may not be as interested in expanding their family, but they often have strong creative and productive urges. They are meant to give birth to something other than physical life (for example, a business or any other form of creative expression).

The third group is in "transition," falling somewhere between the two traditional rhythms of menstruation. This is likely due to external stimuli that have taken us away from our natural flow; for example, current or past use of hormonal birth control, off-kilter circadian rhythms (due to artificial indoor lighting, use of sunglasses when outside, an abundance of illuminated street lights, and the cumulative effect of 24/7 light in larger towns and cities), our increasingly individualistic society, and being unaware of the moon phase. As Griffin states, if you fall into this "transitional" group, it is likely that your body is trying to move toward one of the traditional rhythms of menstruation. "If there were no other influences on our bodies, it would be that way... [But since modern society has so many outside influences], we see a lot of these transitional cycles."[8]

Fascinating, isn't it? After I shared this information with a client, she felt like tracking her cycle and timing her work and life goals around it could be useful. As she stated, "It would help me truly understand and respect my body's needs instead of just drinking extra caffeine or beer to muscle my way through."

I encourage you to begin tracking your cycle if you're not already, and concurrently tracking the phases of the moon. See which group you fall into, and consider the profound impact that nature continues to have on our (still relatively primal) bodies.

To track your monthly cycle and to begin making correlations with your mood (and/or creativity, motivation, etc.) as well as with the cyclical rhythms of the natural world, turn to Appendix A for a "Period, Mood, and Moon Tracker."

For a graphical representation of your monthly cycle, see the image on the following page, which was produced by Jessica Drummond of the Integrative Pelvic Health Institute. For a full-color download of this graphic, go to *www.femfusionfitness.com/images*.

CERVICAL CHANGES DURING YOUR CYCLE

I mentioned the cervical fluid that can be felt during menstruation, but did you know that the uterus (and thus, the cervix) changes position throughout the menstrual cycle? This is not only interesting, but it can also impact sensation for both you and your partner during sex, and it can significantly impact women who suffer from prolapse.

O'Nell Starkey of The Beautiful Cervix Project offers a step-by-step tutorial that will help you get to know your cervix and also confirm where you are in your cycle. As Starkey states, even if you're not charting your menstrual cycles, "have a feel anyway – it's a great skill to have in your empowered woman toolbox!"

The following instructions have been reproduced from www.beautifulcervix.com.

Here's how to feel your cervix:

- *Wash your hands*

- *Squat or stand with one foot raised on a stool.*

- *Insert your longest finger into your vagina until you feel your cervix. It will feel like a protruding nub/cylinder toward the back of the soft walls of your vagina. If your finger is long enough, you should be able to circle your finger all the way around the cervix and feel a little dent in the middle of it (called the os, the opening to the uterus).*

Note the following:

- *How deep in your vagina is your cervix resting? (How much of your finger is inside of you?)*

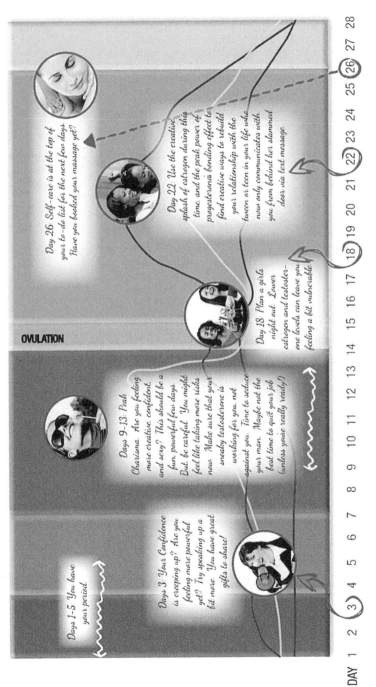

© Jessica Drummond, IPHI

- Does your cervix feel soft, like pursed lips, or firmer, like the tip of your nose?

- Is your cervix angled to one side or aligned more centrally?

- Does your os feel slightly open and squishy or squeezed shut?

While menstruating, the cervix may feel firm and low and the os open as it releases blood. It may be angled to one side slightly. Once all the blood has been shed, the os again feels closed.

As ovulation nears, the rising levels of estrogen cause the ligaments that attach the uterus to the pelvis to tighten and pull the uterus up further into the body. Hence, the cervix gradually draws deeper in the vagina and is often harder to reach near ovulation. The cervix may feel softer (like pursed lips), be more centrally aligned, and the os slightly open.

After ovulation, estrogen levels drop and the cervix usually resumes feeling low, firm, and closed until she gets her period a few weeks later. It is not uncommon for the cervix to be tilted to one side.

Not all women follow this pattern exactly so don't worry if you don't. For example, women with retroverted (tipped) uteruses may find their cervix easier to reach near ovulation and women who have given birth vaginally usually have softer cervices throughout the cycle. It's empowering just to know what is normal for you. You may notice your cervical changes vary from cycle to cycle or that you have a consistent pattern that aligns with your other symptoms of fertility (cervical fluid and basal body temperature).

The key is to check every day so you can feel the relative differences from day to day; cervical changes can be very subtle. Check your cervix in the same position and at the same time each day (i.e. in a squat before showering in the morning), so you're comparing apples to apples – or cervices to cervices, as the case may be.[9]

Chapter 6

THE INNER CORE

We have discussed your external genitalia, your womb, and your menstrual cycle. Now let's get physical and talk about your musculoskeletal system, specifically, your "inner core" (or "deep core" as it is sometimes described). Strengthening your inner core is an essential component to overall health and fitness, but is not always addressed in catchall core fitness programs or "ab-blasting" mat classes.

The inner core is simple to train but there are some basic guidelines that require specific instruction. You need to understand the connection between breath and movement, since the breathing diaphragm marks the "top" of the inner core. You must learn how to properly contract the deep abdominal muscles while maintaining a neutral spine position. You must also learn how to properly engage – and relax – the pelvic floor muscles, which form the base of the inner core.

"Wait a minute…back up. You keep mentioning the pelvic floor. What is the pelvic floor? And why do you keep talking about it?"

Yes, this book focuses heavily on the pelvic floor. Unfortunately, although many women have heard of the pelvic floor, very few are familiar with their own vulvar anatomy, let alone the anatomy of the internal pelvic floor muscles. As we progress from high school health class to our childbearing years and beyond, we are expected to know where the pelvic floor is and what it does. However, since most of us do not receive specific education about this complex region of the body when we are young, we should not be expected to know about it later in life! I didn't know a thing about the pelvic floor until I took extensive anatomy and physiology training in graduate school and saw firsthand where these muscles are and how they function.

Lack of education about our bodies is an unfortunate reality for many women, and it's something I hope to change. When you increase awareness of your deep core muscles (including your pelvic floor) you will be able to isolate and "wake up" your core muscles more effectively. It becomes easier to flatten and tone your stomach, you'll be able to lift and move things safely, and you'll get a better workout each and every time you exercise. The icing on the cake is improved bladder control and increased confidence (and satisfaction) in the bedroom!

The pelvic floor (also known as the PC muscles or "love muscles") is an integral part of your core; you can think if it as the "floor" of your core. Its job is to support the bladder, uterus, and bowels, and to withstand intra-abdominal pressure. It also provides backup bladder and bowel sphincter control, helps with successful delivery of babies, and provides fantastic sensations during orgasm.

MuTu® System (a core fitness program designed for postpartum women) created a fun infographic titled *Fall In Love With Your Pelvic Floor*.[10] This graphic depicts the amusing concept of speed-dating your pelvic floor, describing the pelvic floor's "personality" as:

"Usually a bouncy team player, but without TLC it can become lifeless, tense, and disconnected. Its ambition is to be a useful member of 'Team Core,' to be fit, strong, and functional. Likes regular movement and workouts. Dislikes being ignored... Or permanently clenched."[10]

I love this balanced description almost as much as I love picturing the pelvic floor muscles at a speed-dating event!

If you don't know where your pelvic floor is, you are not alone. Sixty-six percent of women ages 16 and older are unable to locate the pelvic floor, which is a shame since one third of all women experience incontinence (some sources report more), and millions of women suffer pelvic organ prolapse.[11] The pelvic floor is the foundation of the inner core and understanding your pelvic floor anatomy is an essential starting place for the *Lady Bits* program. Whether you cannot yet conceptualize the pelvic floor or you are tired of hearing about the pelvic floor and its importance,

I am here to tell you that you **need** to take the time to **really learn** about this vital region of your body. Keeping it strong and healthy is the key to satisfying sex and control over bodily functions. Yes, I am talking about keeping you dry, keeping you clean, and controlling your gas!

Let's get started. Truly sensing your body, conceptualizing how it works and moves, and understanding your own anatomy is an extremely important component of fitness training.

From top to bottom, the "inner core" includes the:

- Breathing diaphragm
- Deep abdominal and back muscles that surround the trunk
- Pelvic floor muscles

See the following photo for reference:

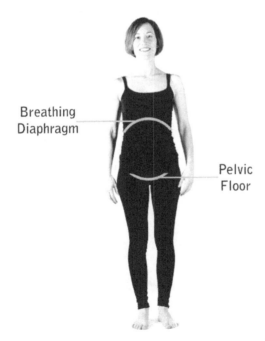

The inner core is difficult to understand because the muscles are deep inside the body. They are just under the skin, not visible like the biceps in the arms, or the rippling "six pack" abdominal muscles (rectus abdominis). Try to **visualize your own inner core** as we run through a brief anatomy lesson.

We will start at the base of the inner core: the pelvic floor.

The pelvic floor consists of a collection of muscles that stretch across the base of the pelvis. To orient yourself, place your hands on the uppermost crests of your pelvis (in other words, "put your hands on your hips"). If you imagine that your hands are on the top edges of a bowl, you can imagine your pelvic floor as the bottom of the bowl.

Let's break down the pelvic floor into its parts. A group of three muscles fan across the base of the pelvis from the pubic bone in the front to the tailbone in the back. These three muscles form what is collectively known as the levator ani. The levator ani provides most of the pelvic floor's mass and power. More superficially (below the levator ani) is a thinner layer of muscles that are collectively known as the urogenital diaphragm. The pelvic floor – including the levator ani and urogenital diaphragm – can be pictured as "the bottom of the bowl" as described above, **or as a hammock** that supports your pelvic organs including your bladder, uterus, and rectum.

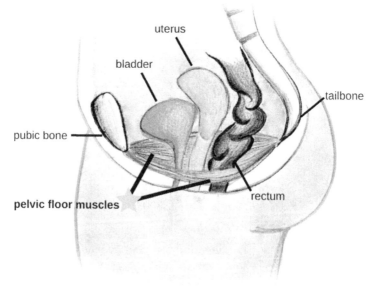

The hammock-like pelvic floor.

In addition to providing hammock-like support, the pelvic floor muscles also surround the urethra, the vagina, and the rectum. When the pelvic floor muscles contract, they contract inward and upward, not only supporting the pelvic organs but also squeezing around urethra, vagina, and rectum. Thus, in addition to holding your organs in place, they help maintain urinary and fecal continence by serving as a closing mechanism along with the urethral and anal sphincters.

Surrounding the pelvic floor are muscles that augment the inner core. Although not part of the "inner core proper," the following muscles provide stability to the pelvis and help to activate the pelvic floor muscles: the hip adductors (brevis, longus, and magnus) and deep hip rotators (obturator internus, piriformis, superior and inferior gemellus, obturator externus, and gluteus minimus).

Moving to the mid-section of the inner core, the deep abdominal and back muscles (including the transversus abdominis, internal and external abdominal obliques, erector spinae, and multifidus) surround the trunk and provide stability to the pelvis and the spine. They help to maintain your posture and alignment. Keeping these hard-working muscles responsive and strong is key when it comes to preventing back pain.

At the very top of the inner core is the breathing diaphragm, an umbrella-shaped muscle that gently moves up and down when you breathe. The diaphragm plays an important role in core stabilization in that it helps to control intra-abdominal pressure and it has an extensive network of fascial (connective tissue) connections to the front, back, and sides of the ribcage and to the spine.

To summarize, the inner core – which is the focus of the physical exercises found in this book – includes the pelvic floor, the deep abdominal muscles, the deep back muscles, and the breathing diaphragm. Remember – understanding your own anatomy is an essential component of fitness training. Improved body awareness begins with education, so let this information really sink in before moving on. If you need to re-read this section, please do so.

Chapter 7

KEGELS: GOOD, BAD, OR INDIFFERENT?

Kegels are the underdog of the exercise world. People don't really like to talk about them, don't like to do them, don't remember to do them, and many don't "get" why they need to do them in the first place! Still others do hundreds of kegels each day, and wonder why their bladder control problems seem to get worse and worse. All of this comes down to a lack of understanding. I will explain, but first let me provide a little background about kegels.

Not everyone knows what a kegel is. Do you? When I asked Mary, 62, to describe how to do a kegel, she said (only half-joking), "First of all, I need to know – **what is a kegel**? It rhymes with bagel... Is it served in a deli?"

"Kegel" is the common name for a pelvic floor isolation exercise in which you **contract and relax** the muscles of the pelvic floor. Kegels are named after Dr. Arnold Kegel, a gynecologist who developed these exercises as a way to help women improve bladder control after surgery and childbirth. Dr. Kegel invented a device called the Perineometer, an instrument that was inserted vaginally to assess the amount of pressure a person could exert with a pelvic floor muscle contraction. He researched the pelvic floor muscles for years, completing multiple studies and working with hundreds of women. His pelvic floor strengthening methods were successful; many patients reported a decrease in urinary incontinence, and as a side effect, women often reported "**enhanced sexual appreciation**." This sparked interest within the fitness world and the world of women, and "kegels" became a buzzword for females who were pregnant and postpartum. Kegels remain an important piece of perinatal education today, although women are rarely specifically educated about when and how to do kegels correctly other than the stern advisory to "do them!"

Dr. Kegel's extensive studies found numerous benefits associated with a program of regular kegels. The following list of benefits is summarized from his breakthrough study, A *Nonsurgical Method of Increasing the Tone of Sphincters and their Supporting Structures*.[12] Dr. Kegel concluded that among patients who did kegels correctly and diligently, the following progressive changes would occur:

- Establishment of **awareness of function** of the pubococcygeus (part of the pelvic floor).

- Slight, gradual increase in Perineometer pressure readings from a level of 1-5 mmHg to as high as 20-40 mmHg or more.

- Muscular contractions felt in areas where none could be demonstrated initially, especially in the anterior and lateral quadrants of the vaginal wall.

- Contractions of the pubococcygeus, which at first were weak and irregular, became strong and sustained.

- Improvement in tone and texture of the tissues of the pelvic floor.

- Increased bulk of the pubococcygeus and its visceral extensions.

- Changes occur in the position of the perineum, introitus (vaginal entrance), urethra, bladder neck, and uterus in relation to an ideal line drawn between the os pubis and coccyx (pelvic bones).

- The vaginal canal became tighter and longer.

- The vaginal walls improved in tone and firmness.

- Bulging of the anterior vaginal wall (often diagnosed as moderate cystocele) became less pronounced.

- Uterine prolapse – when present – usually improved; in some instances the cervix ascended to as high as 5 to 7 cm above the introitus (vaginal opening).

- Supportive pessaries, worn for as long as ten or more years, could usually be discarded without return of discomfort.

- Patients could be fitted with smaller contraceptive diaphragms, whereas diaphragms of larger size formerly slipped out of place.[12]

Despite these awesome findings and the findings of numerous, more recent, studies completed by subsequent researchers, the value of kegels remains controversial. Some practitioners caution all women to avoid isolated pelvic floor strengthening. Among those who promote kegel exercises, there is debate over the exact number of kegels women should complete per exercise session as well as how often kegels should be completed. Some sources encourage hundreds of kegels every day whereas others suggest only five to ten repetitions. Some recommend doing kegels rapidly, others recommend holding the contraction for longer periods of time, and still others recommend a combination approach (both quick and slow-hold kegels)!

To be perfectly honest, the kegel prescription is a mess.

Other controversial issues include whether or not a biofeedback device is required or even helpful for pelvic floor muscle training, whether or not vaginal weights or cones should be used for resistance, and whether or not an examination by a gynecologist, nurse, midwife, or women's health physical therapist is needed to ensure that women are doing kegels correctly. On the last topic, I can tell you with certainty from the literature and from my own experience that many women who think they are doing kegels correctly are not, and an examination from an experienced provider can be very helpful to confirm whether or not you're doing them correctly, and also to determine if they are safe exercises for you to do in the first place.

"But I've heard that kegels are bad…"

I believe that when kegels are "done right" (i.e. when the proper muscles are being isolated, when the pelvic floor is fully relaxed after each contraction), and when they're used within the context of an active lifestyle full of healthy, natural movement, kegels are healthy and beneficial for most (but not all) women. **An active lifestyle is the way nature intended us to move: lots of walking, squatting, lifting, pushing, pulling, and standing/sitting with proper posture, and avoiding excessive sitting (and slouching) on couches or chairs in front of artificially lit screens.** I acknowledge that some women have overly active, tight pelvic floor muscles and for these individuals, kegels should be avoided (keep reading to see if you fall into this category).

I also know that if you are going to do kegels, you must do them responsibly. Make sure you understand how to do kegels correctly and make sure you're balancing your pelvic floor muscles by strengthening the REST of the core muscles as well (the buttocks, hips, abs, back, and breathing diaphragm). The exercises in this book will show you how.

"So kegels aren't bad…but are they necessary?"

Yes AND no. My approach to kegel exercises is BALANCED.

You might be shocked to hear me suggest that kegels may NOT be necessary since I preach the value of core and pelvic floor fitness in my FemFusion® classes, in this book, and on my blog. But just like most things in life, there are two sides to the kegel story, and the following point deserves driving home: **MOVEMENT is necessary. Kegels are not (necessarily) necessary.**

All movement relies on the core and pelvic floor to provide stability and control, so if you walk, squat, jump, pull, push, lunge, and rotate regularly, you'll naturally be toning and using these essential muscles all day long.

As biomechanist Katy Bowman says, pelvic floor health depends on natural movement (i.e. walking, squatting, kneeling, lifting, changing positions) done throughout the day. She calls this "movement nutrition," stating that how we move – and the quantity and quality of our movement – is just as important as the foods we put into our body when it comes to health and wellness.[13] In fact, the very act of movement helps us assimilate the nutrients we receive via food. Movement stimulates blood flow to circulate and help us utilize the nutrients we consume, and the load that we put on our bones and joints helps us build and maintain bone density (again, allowing us to properly utilize the nutrients we ingest).

Check in with yourself: Are you getting enough "movement nutrition?" Is your body hungry for more?

If we lived in an ideal society, moving in the ways – and in the quantities – that humans were designed to move, then our pelvic floor muscles would naturally be kept supple, vital, and strong. Here are some examples of this ideal "utopian" society (as far as movement is concerned). We would be:

- Moving regularly throughout the day. Changing positions often – bending, squatting, standing, sitting, walking, etc.

- Performing manual labor and ACTIVE activities of daily living – working in the garden, hunting or gathering food, cleaning and maintaining the home without the use of modern technology.

- Squatting when using the restroom.

- Lifting, pushing, and pulling objects of all sizes – heavy, and lightweight.

- Walking, running, actively playing with our children...simply MOVING MORE without being tethered to modern technology that tends to keep us motionless and fixated on our device.

- Giving birth naturally, when our bodies are ready, without modern medical intervention such as episiotomy and/or synthetic oxytocin (which can be medically necessary and even life-saving, but is arguably over-utilized in modern society).

- Living life unencumbered by excess body weight or obesity, which contributes to pressure and strain on the muscles of the core and pelvic floor.

If we lived and moved in these ways, most women would retain well-functioning pelvic floor muscles (not to mention the rest of the body) into old age. We would be less likely to develop pelvic organ prolapse. **We would be in control of our bladders!** We would retain the natural reflexes that cause the pelvic floor muscles to assist the urethral and anal sphincters by reflexively contracting before a cough or a sneeze to help keep us dry and leak-free.

We would NOT need to do kegels!

Unfortunately, for most modern women – due to a largely sedentary lifestyle (leading to muscular disuse) and/or trauma during childbirth – we lose these natural pelvic floor reflexes over time. We also lose vitality in the muscles of the core and the pelvic floor leading to lack of sensation and responsiveness during sex.

I do think that a shift in consciousness is happening. Most people today acknowledge and understand the importance of exercise and MOVEMENT in terms of health benefits, and more and more people are interested in adopting a healthy, active lifestyle. But is the message taking hold? Is it being implemented? Are people really doing it? Not enough. **We're not quite "there."** Thus, for many modern women, kegels are helpful when part of a balanced core strengthening program.

The truth about kegels is that they are an important component of inner core fitness for many women today. However, the goal should not be to complete hundreds of kegels just for the sake of creating a strong pelvic floor. Rather, the goal should be to practice kegels regularly enough to ensure that the pelvic floor muscles can be activated quickly and effectively when needed. A secondary – but no less important – goal is to gain sufficient stamina for everyday activities that require pelvic floor muscle activation.

What types of everyday activities require pelvic floor muscle activation? Too many to list! The following is a sample of common situations that have challenged my (and my friends' and clients') pelvic floor strength. When you can activate your pelvic floor muscles quickly and effectively, you will be able to:

- Hold your bladder during a long car ride when there is no rest area in sight.

- Join your kids or grandchildren on the trampoline without needing to change your underwear afterward.

- Prevent urinary leakage by "bracing" with a pelvic floor contraction before you cough or sneeze.

- Make it to the bathroom on time when you **really have to go!**

- Avoid leakage when laughter threatens to make you the butt of the old joke, "I laughed so hard tears ran down my legs."

- Carry a heavy box up or down stairs while maintaining core stability (and dry underwear).

- Maintain continence when you have to sprint across the street to catch a cab or when you are pulled across the park as your dog chases a squirrel.

- Live a life unencumbered by low back pain (pelvic floor and core weakness can contribute to spinal instability and back problems).

- Feel confident that you have the strength, stamina, and coordination to use your pelvic floor muscles to enhance sexual pleasure.

It is vitally important to acknowledge the importance of pelvic floor muscle **coordination**. I often hear women complain that they do kegel exercises every day without relief from incontinence. When I inform these women that the key to pelvic floor fitness is not just how strong the muscles are but how quickly and easily they can **use them when they need them** (coordination), a light bulb moment occurs and they say, "Oh! Now I get it!"

It all boils down to understanding and connecting to your own pelvic floor. In the medical world, we call this "neuromuscular reeducation," but in real life we just call it "connection."

"I'm a modern woman… I know I sit too much. So I'll just do a few kegels and then I'll be fine?"

No. As you proceed with this or any other core strengthening program that promotes inner core and pelvic floor wellness, keep in mind that kegels – on their own – are only part of the story when it comes to treating incontinence, preventing prolapse, revving up your sex drive, and improving back pain and balance. A comprehensive pelvic floor fitness program includes exercises for all of the muscles of the inner core (including the pelvic floor, deep back and abdominal muscles, and the diaphragm) and pelvic girdle (including the gluteals, adductors, and hip rotators). **In order for the pelvic floor to work optimally, it must be surrounded and supported by strong muscles!** A well-rounded program teaches you how to maintain strength and flexibility of all of these muscles, and most importantly, teaches you how to use the muscles appropriately.

WHO SHOULD AVOID KEGELS

Some women hold chronic tension in their pelvic floor and their muscles are short and tight most of the day. This often results in pain with intercourse, difficulty initiating urination, and a feeling of tension or pain in the pelvic area. If this describes you, discontinue any attempts at kegels. Feel free to practice Core Breathing (Chapter 11) and the relaxation exercises found in Chapter 21, but do not focus on kegels or isolated pelvic floor strengthening until you have consulted with a women's health physical therapist.

Even if you don't have any sensation of pain or tension in the pelvic region, if you think you're doing kegels correctly but still aren't seeing results, seek the care of a women's health physical therapist. She can help you troubleshoot and determine an appropriate pelvic floor strengthening (or relaxation/down-training) program based on your individual needs.

> "Once we accept our limits, we go beyond them."
> –Albert Einstein

FOCUS ON TECHNIQUE

Contracting and relaxing the pelvic floor muscles may seem simple, but surprisingly, many women who think they know how to do a kegel are not utilizing the appropriate muscles when examined for technique. There are a few steps you must take to make sure you are "kegeling" correctly. If you are not completing kegels correctly, your strengthening efforts will be ineffective and you may actually be stressing your pelvic floor.

EXERCISE – Correct Kegels:

Lie on your back with a pillow under your hips and your knees bent (see picture). Place a hand on your belly and breathe normally. Contract your pelvic floor muscles – the "bottom of the bowl," or the hammock that sits at the base of your pelvis – by <u>squeezing and lifting</u> the muscles as if you are trying to stop the flow of urine. You can also imagine that you are pulling a marble into your vagina and up toward your bellybutton. I know it sounds strange, but this is a great way to describe what the contraction portion of a kegel feels like.

Now for the most important part: <u>fully relax the pelvic floor muscles.</u> Completely let go. If you imagined pulling a marble into your vagina, relax by mentally allowing the marble to roll out.

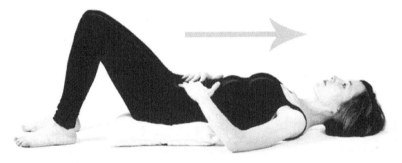

Ask yourself some questions. Did your pelvic floor move downward when you tried to contract? Did you feel your buttocks clenching? Were you holding your breath? Were you bearing down, as if to have a bowel movement? Did your belly distend outward, or draw in strongly? Do you feel like your pelvic floor muscles are still tense? If you answered yes to any of these questions, then you did not do the kegel correctly. The aim of a kegel is to isolate the pelvic floor muscles with just a tiny bit of help (co-contraction) from the surrounding muscles such as the transverse abdominis (one of the deep abdominal muscles). **Remember – the primary**

movement comes from the pelvic floor muscles, not the buttocks or the abs. Also recall that the pelvic floor muscles are internal, so there should be no significant external movement as they contract and relax.

Ready for the next step? This is another way to tune into your body and improve control and coordination of the pelvic floor. Recall that the pelvic floor muscles encircle three openings: the urethra in the front, the vagina in the middle, and the anus in the back. Use your body awareness – your "internal compass" – to locate and connect with the three zones of your pelvic floor. Although subtle, it is absolutely possible to differentiate between the three zones and to isolate each zone when you contract. Practice engaging the muscles around each opening separately **without clenching your buttocks or tucking your tailbone under**. Focus your attention around the anus and think of stopping wind or gas; close the opening, then lift up and in. Next, focus on the vagina and/or urethra; close the opening(s), and then lift. As before, be sure to relax fully after each contraction.

COME ON, TAKE A LOOK!

Here I go again... You need to know your own anatomy better than your partner does! Grab a mirror and take a look.

To make sure you are performing kegels correctly, use a handheld mirror as you lie in the position described above. This is best done without underwear. As you contract the pelvic floor, the perineum – the area between the vagina and the anus – should move upward and inward (toward your head). **This is a tiny movement.** If you see the perineum bulging outward, stop here! You are not doing a kegel correctly. Read on for more information and then try again. As you relax the pelvic floor, the perineum should move slightly downward, back to its natural resting position.

In addition to looking, do not be afraid to **touch**! This is your body... You need to **know it**.

Lightly touch the perineum (the area between the vagina and the anus) while you perform the kegel. This can be done with or without underwear. Again, you should feel the perineum move upward (toward your head) as you contract, and downward (toward your feet) as you relax. This is a very small movement. If the perineum does not move or if it bulges downward *as you contract*, stop here and keep reading for more tips before trying again.

I highly encourage you to move on to the next level, and actually insert your finger into the vaginal canal to really get a sense of where the pelvic floor muscles are, and how they feel when you're performing a kegel. After you've inserted your (clean) finger, possibly lubricated for comfort, perform a kegel. You should feel the muscles surrounding the vagina gently clamp "in and up" around your finger. Note the strength of the contraction. Was it a tiny movement? Or was it strong, like a baby sucking? Were you able to feel both the contraction and the relaxation phase? The goal is to feel both a distinct contraction AND relaxation of the pelvic floor.

Another technique involving tactile sensory input that can be very effective is the following: lightly sit (straddle) the arm of a sturdy chair. Feel the surface of the chair lightly touching your perineum. Now squeeze and lift your pelvic floor muscles in an attempt to lift the skin of your perineum **away from** the arm of the chair. You should feel the perineum move upward (toward your head) as you contract, and downward (back toward the arm of the chair) as you relax. Again, if it does not move or if it bulges downward *as you contract*, stop here and keep reading for more tips before trying again.

The above techniques – looking and touching – are called "simple biofeedback." They provide sensory information (visual and tactile) to the brain to help coordinate the command with the movement.

If you are not able to perform a kegel correctly, try concentrating on the following visualizations. After you have found one that makes sense to you or resonates with you, try the exercise again with one of the simple biofeedback techniques described above.

Visualization One: The Flower. Think of your vagina as a flower that is wide open, like a rose in full bloom. Contract your pelvic floor muscles (pull them inward and upward) as you visualize the flower closing up tightly into a bud, like time-lapse photography going backward from summer to spring. Relax the pelvic floor as you visualize the flower once again in full bloom.

Visualization Two: The Elevator. This is my favorite visualization for kegels. Imagine your pelvic floor muscles as an elevator that is stopped at the ground floor or the lobby of a building. Contract your pelvic floor muscles as you imagine the elevator doors sliding closed, and then lift your pelvic floor muscles upward as you imagine the elevator rising to the second or third floor. Hold briefly at the top of the contraction. Release the contraction as the imaginary elevator lowers and returns to the starting position (the lobby). Fully relax your pelvic floor muscles as you imagine the elevator doors sliding open.

Visualization Three: The Door. Imagine your vagina as a door that is wide open, letting in light. Visualize the door closing shut as you contract your pelvic floor muscles (pull them inward and upward). Think of the darkness. Then visualize the door swinging wide open and letting the light back in as you relax the pelvic floor muscles.

Visualization Four: The String. Imagine a string that is tied to your perineum and runs up through your bellybutton. Imagine pulling the string upward (toward your head) out of your bellybutton as you contract your pelvic floor muscles. Then imagine letting go of the string as you relax the pelvic floor.

Visualization Five: The Silk Handkerchief. Imagine there's a silk handkerchief directly underneath your vagina. Draw the middle of the imaginary hankie into your vagina as if you're tenting it and pulling it into your body. Then release it; drop it gently back down, and imagine it fluttering to the floor. NOTE: This works best in squatting, sitting on your heels with your knees slightly apart, or standing.

Visualization Six: The Marble. Breathe deeply into the back of your rib cage, then exhale as you lift your pelvic floor as if picking up a marble with your vagina, or drawing a tampon up inside you. Then release, and visualize the marble rolling out of your body as you relax the pelvic floor muscles.

Fun Tidbit: Don't kegel when you pee! At some point in the history of "kegeling," word got out that women should do kegels while urinating. THIS IS NOT TRUE. The logic behind this theory is that since you use your pelvic floor muscles to voluntarily stop the flow of urine, if you can stop your urine stream, you'll know whether or not you can successfully contract and relax your pelvic floor muscles. Here's the deal – it's okay to try a kegel or two while you urinate in order to "check in" to see if you are doing kegels correctly (to see if you can stop and re-start the flow of urine), **but this is not something you should do on a regular basis**. Regularly doing kegels while urinating can lead to incomplete bladder evacuation, which can make your bladder feel like it's always full. You might think your bladder is the size of an acorn, but in reality, it's simply never fully empty! To fully empty your bladder, practice your kegel exercises when you are OFF the toilet.

Also, many women tell me that they do kegels when driving. That's fine – as long as you can fully sense both the pelvic floor muscle contraction and relaxation *while also concentrating on the road*. I find that when I do kegels while driving, something suffers. Either I am not fully concentrating on my kegels (and therefore largely wasting my time by doing half-hearted contractions), or I do concentrate on the kegels, which causes my mind to wander from the road. My speed slows, my car starts to weave a bit in traffic – not a safe situation! I realize that multi-tasking is appealing; however, focus is important for effective kegels and for safe driving. I do kegels professionally and I still need to concentrate... My guess is that you do, too.

PUTTING IT INTO PRACTICE: KEGEL VARIATIONS

We just spent several pages ensuring that you can successfully isolate the muscles of the pelvic floor. My hope is that you read through the instructions for completing a pelvic floor muscle contraction – or kegel – in the section titled, "Focus on Technique." If you have not done that yet, please return to that section and read it now.

Let's discuss some practical kegel variations. Quick kegels are important to practice so that you will be able to quickly utilize the pelvic floor muscles when you need them, for example, to prepare for a cough or sneeze. The slow-hold (endurance) kegels are important for situations that require longer periods of pelvic floor muscle activation, such as jumping on a trampoline, running, or maintaining your balance – for example, during "tree pose" in a yoga class or when you are standing at the top of a ladder.

Although the *Lady Bits* program does not require you to do kegels every day, quick and endurance kegels are incorporated into the Inner Core Energizer routine. And in Chapter 21, I describe how to use kegels during sex. Think of this kegel practice session as an introduction to things to come! Give it a try.

EXERCISE – Quick and Endurance Kegels:

Lie down and take a personal assessment of your own pelvic floor strength. Complete one to three quick kegels, just as a check-in. If you are able to feel a strong contraction and full relaxation when you are lying down, progress to an upright position such as seated or standing. When upright (sitting or standing), you are contracting your pelvic floor muscles against gravity. This is more challenging for your pelvic floor but it will give you a better feel for how well you can use your pelvic floor muscles in the "real world," since your waking hours are generally spent upright. If you have difficulty sensing your pelvic floor muscle contractions or feel that your pelvic floor muscles are weak, do not progress to an upright position at this time; rather, continue to lie down.

Now for the kegels! For quick kegels, quickly contract (squeeze and lift) the pelvic floor, and then fully relax. Feel as if you are pulling an imaginary marble into your vagina when contracting, then let the marble roll out of your vagina when relaxing. Alternatively, you may use any of the visualizations already discussed. Complete 10 quick kegels.

For endurance kegels, contract (squeeze and lift) the pelvic floor and hold for 8-10 seconds, and then fully relax the pelvic floor. Again, you can use the marble visualization or any other visualization technique that works well for you. Complete 5 to 10 repetitions of endurance kegels, being sure to fully relax between each rep.

This is just practice; it is not something that you need to do every day, as long as you are getting plenty of movement and regularly completing the upcoming Inner Core Energizer routine.

The key is **not** to do kegels all day long, every day, simply to make the pelvic floor muscles strong. **Productivity is not the goal**. Instead, the goals are:

- To practice kegels with **purpose and awareness** so you know how to activate (and relax) your pelvic floor muscles when that little "extra" is needed (neuromuscular reeducation).

- To understand how to use your pelvic floor muscles to support certain movements and exercises (proper body mechanics).

- To gain stamina for everyday activities since the pelvic floor is always "on" – albeit at a low level of muscular activation.

ONE MORE CHECK-IN

As a reminder, the following are cues that you are NOT performing a kegel correctly:

- You can feel or see your buttocks clenching.

- Your abdominals are bulging outward or strongly pulling inward (i.e. your abdominals are working harder than your pelvic floor).

- You find yourself holding your breath.

- You are pushing or bearing down.

- Your symptoms (such as incontinence, prolapse, or pain) are getting worse, not better.

Please do not be discouraged if it takes some time to "get the hang of it." Up to fifty percent of women are unable to complete kegels correctly with verbal or written instruction alone. If you feel that this is the case for you, seek out a women's health physical therapist, nurse midwife, gynecologist, or urogynecologist. These healthcare providers have special training in the treatment of pelvic floor dysfunction including underactive, overactive, or poorly coordinated pelvic floor muscles. They can help you locate your pelvic floor muscles and find a pelvic floor strengthening (or relaxation) program based on your strength level and your specific needs. In time, you can return to this book to augment the program they have provided.

Chapter 8

BODY MECHANICS AND POSTURE: TOOLS FOR LIFE

In the following sections, I will describe some everyday situations that require you to effectively engage your pelvic floor muscles in order to maintain bodily control and stability. Got back pain? You need to read this.

"ZIPPING UP" FOR POSTURE AND STABILITY

When people try to improve their posture, often they focus on the abdominal muscles. They stand tall and suck in their tummies. However, in order to fully (and safely) engage the muscles of the core to maximize stability and control, you need to start at the base of your inner core – the pelvic floor – and then work your way up. "**Zipping up**" is a cornerstone of the Inner Core Energizer routine, and is essential for female athletes who lift weights.

EXERCISE – Zipping Up:

First, focus on your posture. Stand with your feet hip-width apart and toes pointing forward, shoulders relaxed, arms at your sides.

Find your neutral spine position. There should be a gentle inward curve in your lower (lumbar) spine. Be sure that your low back isn't flattened and that your tailbone isn't tucked under. Avoid the "long-butt" look! On the flipside, you also want to avoid an overly exaggerated lumbar curve (i.e. a "swayback" look, or a gymnast's stance).

Rotate your arms and hands so that your thumbs face outward (away from your body) – this will gently engage the muscles between your shoulder blades.

When you do this, be sure that your low back doesn't arch and that your lower ribs don't pop forward.

Now relax your arms and hands so that your palms face inward, toward your body.

Next, visualize a zipper that starts (fastens) at your vagina.

Begin "zipping up" by gently squeezing and lifting the pelvic floor (do a gentle kegel). The effort you put into this kegel should be similar to the pressure you would apply to test an avocado for ripeness – gentle! Do not clench or grip the pelvic floor muscles.

Next, imagine drawing the "zipper" upward as you engage the abdominals. Think of the lowest, deepest band of abdominal muscles, just above your pubic bone. Draw this region gently inward and upward, toward your head. I liken this "in and up" sensation to the feeling of fastening a snug pair of jeans.

As you zip up, stand tall and feel the crown of your head drawing up toward the ceiling. When fully zipped, make sure your forehead is soft and relaxed, and then check in with your shoulders once again. Relax your shoulders downward if tension has drawn them upward. Be sure that your shoulder blades are drawn gently down and back, and make sure that your weight is distributed evenly over your feet.

Remember, engaging the inner core muscles in this manner should not feel like "clenching." Hyper-activation of any muscle group can lead to pain and ultimately weakness due to muscle fatigue. Painful trigger points can develop, and if the gluteal and abdominal muscles become overactive they can pull your pelvis into a position called posterior pelvic tilt. This creates a posture in which your back loses the normal curvature at the lumbar spine; your back flattens and your bottom tucks under. Avoid this position – it is unhealthy for your spine (and is unflattering, too)!

"Do I need to 'zip up' all day long?"

No. Regarding inner core muscle activation, a fine balance needs to be established.

When sedentary, the inner core muscles should be as relaxed as possible while maintaining a neutral spine position (in other words, while maintaining proper posture and alignment). When your spine and pelvis are in a neutral position, all of your core muscles are at the perfect length and tension to support your body, and crucially, to quickly and effectively fire on demand. As stated by Tasha Mulligan, physical therapist and founder of the Hab-it system for pelvic floor fitness, "[proper] positioning of our pelvis allows our muscles to fire when they need to fire, and when they are 'resting' they are held in a position of light tension that leaves them ready to work the instant they are called upon again."[14]

However, you should consciously "zip up" when preparing to complete something strenuous. Examples include vacuuming, lifting weights, lifting a laundry basket, or simply bending forward to get a file out of a filing cabinet. In these situations, you must understand how to "extra-engage" the inner core muscles by **zipping**. You will feel lifted, strong, secure, and – most importantly – you will be protected from injury.

THE PELVIC BRACE TECHNIQUE

"I've been feeling a lot of pressure in the vaginal area recently. I'm not sure what's going on, but each time I cough, I feel like something inside my body presses down into the vagina. I feel like it's getting worse! What's happening?"

Have you ever felt this sensation? If so, it's possible that you have developed pelvic organ prolapse. Whether you have prolapse or stress incontinence – or don't have either, but want to prevent them from occurring in the future – you need to learn (and utilize) the pelvic brace technique. The pelvic brace, also known as "the knack," is a preemptive tightening of the pelvic floor muscles prior to activities that create an increase in intra-abdominal pressure.

Remember this helpful phrase: "Squeeze before you sneeze" (and cough, and blow your nose, and lift, and blow up a balloon, and laugh)... In short, contract your pelvic floor muscles any time you anticipate a significant amount of downward pressure on the pelvic floor. The pelvic brace helps support the pelvic organs from below, thereby preventing risk of prolapse or bladder leakage.

The pelvic brace is a reflexive action; however, many women lose it over the course of time, which often includes childbirth, surgeries, weight gain, and so on. Ultimately, women who have lost the pelvic brace reflex need to practice the pelvic brace technique in order to re-train their muscles.

The following describes how to do the pelvic brace technique. Give it a try right now and see how it feels. If it feels foreign or awkward, I recommend practicing the technique three to five times on a regular basis in order to make the pelvic brace a habit – a part of your "muscle memory." This will keep you dry when you cough or sneeze and will help prevent the progression of pelvic organ prolapse.

EXERCISE – Pelvic Brace:

Strongly squeeze and lift the pelvic floor (do a kegel). <u>Hold</u> the contraction, and then gently cough.

After the cough is complete, relax the pelvic floor muscles fully.

Repeat if desired. Get in the habit of preparing for a cough, sneeze, or nose-blow by utilizing the pelvic brace technique.

EXHALE ON EXERTION

Women's wellness guru and perinatal fitness expert Jenny Burrell is famous for her phrase, "exhale on exertion."[15]

As Burrell states, "MOMS LIFT STUFF! All blooming day long, they're lifting and 'loading' their bodies against gravity."[15] Lifting creates a natural increase in intra-abdominal pressure, which forces your internal organs downward and outward. This is a significant problem if your abdominal wall and/or your pelvic floor muscles are weak. Repetitive lifting with improper breathing mechanics can result in a stubborn tummy pooch or problems with urinary leakage.

The solution is simple. As you lift yourself, your baby, your dog, your groceries, a barbell, or anything else – as you rise against gravity, **exhale on exertion**!

Why does exhaling on exertion help? Because a lot happens when you exhale. Your diaphragm rises, the pressure in your abdomen decreases, your pelvic floor muscles naturally lift, and your deep abdominal muscles naturally engage. Do it right now and see. As you exhale you should feel an automatic tensioning (activation) of your deep inner core muscles. Isn't it fantastic how everything works together?

It might take some retraining, but it's well worth the effort. Practice "exhaling on exertion," and in time it will become automatic.

A PRIMER ON POSTURE

I know, I know...you've heard it before. Good posture is important. I already addressed it, so why belabor the subject?

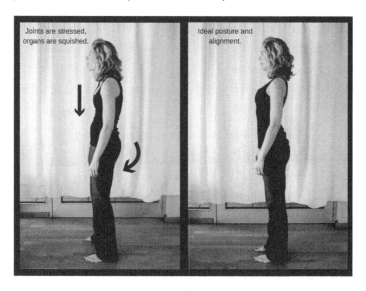

In a nushell, bad posture = big problems. Your body doesn't exist in single, isolated segments. In the spirit of the classic folk song "Dem Bones," we're all just big long chains of body parts from our toe bones to our head bone. One area affects the next, which affects the next, which affects the next, and so on. When your posture or alignment is "off" in any one area, from your ankles (when you wear high heels) to your spine (when you slouch), to your neck (when you jut your head forward to squint at a computer screen), you will feel it. If not now, then you will feel it a few months or years from now. Even mild postural problems can affect your health.

Standing (or sitting) with poor posture puts excessive pressure on your abdominal and pelvic organs and strains the muscles and connective tissues surrounding your joints. Here are some of the not-so-fun issues that can result from poor posture:

- A poochy tummy – and even diastasis recti (more on this later) – from your abdominal contents being pushed forward/outward.

- Pelvic organ prolapse from your pelvic organs (bladder, rectum, uterus) being pushed downward. The structure of your bony pelvis prevents downward descent of the pelvic organs when your pelvis is in the correct position, but when your pelvis is NOT in the correct position – when it is tipped back (posterior tilt, as seen in the photo at left above) – the pelvic organs can descend through the space that makes the birthing canal. If you have a dysfunctional pelvic floor to boot, you're almost guaranteed to develop pelvic organ prolapse at some point in your life.

- Constant pressure on the bladder and bowels due to your abdominal and pelvic contents being "squished" because of poor posture. This can lead to feelings of urinary and fecal urgency and bladder control issues.

- Musculoskeletal problems including hip and low back pain, upper back pain, neck pain...the works.

You MUST align your body, get out of high heeled shoes, sit less, and untuck your tailbone to enable your pelvic floor muscles to work optimally and at their ideal length.

Good posture isn't complicated, but it takes practice and frequent check-ins to make sure you've got it right. **Even if you practiced this during the "zipping" exercise, do it again. Right now.**

EXERCISE – Proper Posture:

Stand with your feet and knees pointing straight ahead. Your feet should be hip-width apart, toes pointed forward.

Allow your pelvis to be in a neutral position so that your low back isn't overly-arched or super-flat. If you're accustomed to tucking your tailbone under (often unconsciously done as a way to minimize the appearance of your derrière), you might feel like you're sticking your bottom out. You're probably not. Take a look in the mirror to be sure.

Roll your shoulders up, and then down and back, so that your shoulders are down and away from your ears and your chest is open.

When you do this, be sure that your low back doesn't excessively arch and that your lower ribs don't pop forward. If they do, gently pull your lower ribs inward and return your spine to a neutral position.

Lift the crown of your head up toward the ceiling, making sure that your forehead and face are relaxed.

You should be standing tall, in perfect alignment with your head over your hips over your heels.

"That's how to stand...but how should I sit?"

When sitting, sit on your sit bones (your "butt bones," or in proper anatomical terms, your ischial tuberosities) with your spine, shoulders, and head in alignment as noted above. Please do not slouch and sit on your sacrum or your tailbone! This can lead to back pain and "squishing" of your internal organs as previously described.

Tomorrow, plan to do regular posture checks throughout the day. Every hour, on the hour, take a moment to notice how you're sitting, standing, or walking. These impromptu "posture checks" will reveal how you typically hold your body throughout the day. If your posture looks good, move on! If it needs some work, take a few days to really focus on finding (and maintaining) proper alignment. Your bones, joints, and pelvic organs will thank you.

"I get it – posture is important. But I'm still hung up on the fact that you mentioned 'getting out of high heels.' What?! Why?!"

Yep...you read correctly! I'm a firm believer in balance, and I think that the occasional use of high heels for an evening out is fine, but if you wear heels daily – even low heels – you are doing your body a disservice.

You have roughly 200 bones in your entire body, and 25% of them reside from the ankles down.[16] Furthermore, about a quarter of all the muscles and motor nerves in your body are dedicated to your feet! Cramming your feet and toes into a stiff and unreasonably narrow shoe – and then adding a heel to it – is unnatural and ultimately unsafe for your body.

Why? Because as biomechanist Katy Bowman explains, geometry matters. She states, "Although the height of [even] a short heel may just be one or two inches, the foot is relatively short in length compared to

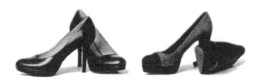

Lady Bits

the height of the body, so the number of degrees that a one- or two-inch heel can displace you is quite large."[16] Just think of those five-inch stilettos that some women wear!

Bowman goes on to state that the higher the heel, the greater you will (unconsciously) compensate by shifting your posture. She explains, "A person can compensate for the high, forward pitch with their ankles, knees, pelvic tilt, or spinal curvature. Any one of these joints can be displaced to make the heel wearer look fairly upright, even if their bones are not truly vertical or loaded optimally."[16]

Aside from the whole body displacement, which changes the loading on the bones and joints and the length-tension relationship of the muscles (such as the pelvic floor), wearing heels also increases the load on the front of the foot, potentially leading to circulatory issues and even bunions.

So other than a few hours on your anniversary, get out of those heels. The long-limbed look is just not worth the long-term consequences. For more detail on this subject, I highly recommend Bowman's book, *Every Woman's Guide to Foot Pain Relief: The New Science of Healthy Feet*.

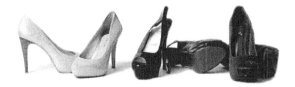 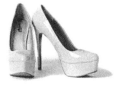

PART III:
Real Life Lessons in Radiant Aging

THE ONLY THING CONSTANT IS CHANGE.

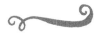

"A woman's health is her capital."
–Harriet Beecher Stowe

"I am not young but I feel young. The day I feel old, I will go to bed and stay there. J'aime la vie! I feel that to live is a wonderful thing."
–Coco Chanel

"Life really does begin at forty. Up until then, you are just doing research."
–Carl Jung

Chapter 9

WHAT TO EXPECT AS YOU AGE

We're going to spend some time on this. In order to really get to know, love, and accept yourself, you need to understand your body and what's going on (or what will go on in the future) so that you can be mentally and physically prepared for the changes ahead. No matter your age, you will benefit from reading and absorbing this section.

Please note that the following list of changes is NOT exhaustive or all-inclusive. I will not delve deeply into prenatal or postpartum issues – that's another book in and of itself! Nor will I delve into specifics when it comes to hormone imbalances, specific disease processes, and all the many possible variations among women. Rather, I intend to present an overview of some of the common changes that many women will encounter over the course of their lifetimes; little "bits" of information that are – or will be – relevant to you.

The topics ahead focus on general lifestyle and musculoskeletal problems, which are my areas of expertise, and within my scope of practice. I provide resources for further reading if you want to dig a little deeper. I'll also provide plenty of real-life stories from friends, clients, and my own personal experiences. So pour yourself a cup of tea and get ready to learn.

KAREN'S STORY

The following is from Karen, one of the original participants in my FemFusion® group exercise classes. Karen found that focusing on the inner core during her workouts made a huge difference in terms of urinary control and overall body confidence.

On baby weight:

"I didn't notice any significant changes in my body after my first baby. I was in decent shape and I 'bounced back.' It was my second baby that really impacted my body. I remember seeing these huge thighs, cellulite dimples and all! I thought, 'whose thighs are these?' I also noticed a double chin I had never had before. I didn't see it coming... It startled me!

I was able to get most of the extra weight off after my second child was born, but I had to work a lot harder. I could not simply rely on nature to return me to my former skinny self. For the person who had always been the skinniest girl in the room without even trying, this was a big blow."

On urinary incontinence:

"Sneezing in public is awful. I am a serious career woman and I think of myself as being 'in control' of everything, so why is it that when I sneeze I have to cross my legs or I'll wet my pants? It's just not fair! The bladder leakage is completely involuntary, and I hate it. If I can't even control my pee, then what can I control?"

You may find your own symptoms reflected in Karen's story. Retention of baby weight, pelvic organ prolapse, and involuntary bladder leakage are legitimate – and common – concerns that many women deal with but few women openly discuss. I am doing my best to change that! I encourage dialogue about issues that are common among women so that no one feels alone or "weird" about changes they encounter. As you read, consider:

Which of these changes have I gone through?
Which of these changes do I fear?
Which of these have I dismissed or condemned in other people?
Which of these do I recognize in a family member or friend?

PREGNANCY AND CHILDBIRTH

Pregnancy is something that many women experience one or more times and it has profound effects on the body, mind, and spirit. For now, we'll focus on the body.

Changes occur in the inner core early in pregnancy with a decrease in pelvic floor muscular activity noted as early as the eighth week gestation.[17] Many women begin having incontinence issues for the first time in their lives when they are pregnant, which can come as quite a surprise! Urinary leakage can occur due to the weight of the baby creating a downward force on the pelvic floor muscles, which are stretched – sometimes to the max – during the course of pregnancy. When the pelvic floor muscles are overstretched, they can't effectively help close off the urethra. This can cause spontaneous leakage of urine, for example, while walking or during activities that cause an increase in intra-abdominal pressure such as lifting, moving from sit to stand, and coughing or laughing.

In addition to the pelvic floor changes, the abdominal muscles become stretched during pregnancy, sometimes creating a diastasis – or separation – of the rectus abdominis (the "six pack" muscles). This is a reversible condition, but takes extra care during postpartum exercise rehabilitation. Let's take a closer look at diastasis recti.

DIASTASIS RECTI

Two out of three women experience a separation of the abdominal muscles – called diastasis recti (DR) – during their pregnancy. When the abdominal muscles separate, the linea alba – the connective tissue that joins the muscles together – stretches sideways and becomes thin and weak. Some separation is normal and quickly reverses on its own, but a larger separation takes time and special care to close.

Many women aren't aware that they have DR until well after delivery, or even after their baby has become a toddler, when they develop an abdominal hernia, chronic low back pain, or they just can't get rid of the "mommy tummy." All of these problems can occur due to an unclosed diastasis. The lingering "mommy tummy" may actually be partially due to protruding abdominal organs. One of the functions of the abdominal muscles – besides supporting your posture, providing spinal stability, and preventing low back pain – is to compress your abdominal contents and keep everything in place. If you have an unclosed diastasis, your abs aren't able to compress your abdominal contents the way they did before the separation.

Even if you had your baby YEARS ago, you can (and should) check yourself for DR. The following self-check steps are from Jenny Burrell, a women's wellness expert who teaches health and fitness professionals holistic methods for healing DR.[18]

EXERCISE – DR Self-Check:

Lie on your back with your knees bent, and your feet flat on the floor.

Place one hand behind your head to support its weight and lift your shoulder blades 1-2 inches off the floor. This creates an increase in intra-abdominal pressure and a contraction of the rectus abdominis (RA) muscles that will allow you to measure the gap between the two bellies of the RA and check the tension of the midline connective tissues (the linea alba).

As you perform this mini-lift, use your free hand to assess whether or not you have DR. Here's how:

- *Hold your index and middle finger of your free hand together and vertical. Starting at the softness just below the bottom of your ribcage, directly in the middle of your tummy, feel width-ways across your RA muscles. Start at the top and feel all the way down to your belly button and then beyond to your bikini line.*

- *What you're looking for: First, how many fingers fit into the gap of the "gully" between the strips of the RA muscles the full length of your abdomen? Second, how much tension is there in the linea alba? How much resistance is there to your fingers?*

- *A gap or "gully" into which your fingers descend without*

*much resistance is considered to be POSITIVE FOR
DIASTASIS RECTI. If this is found, traditional abdominal
exercises such as "crunches" should be avoided until either
the gap has closed OR more importantly, the midline
tissues have regained a degree of tension that withstands
the pressure of your finger pressure and ultimately the
level of exercise that you seek to do. It is important to
understand that for many women, the gap might not close
fully, but regaining sufficient tension through the entire
abdominal wall and at the midline can be sufficient to
create a "functional diastasis" where the woman looks and
feels well, and doesn't suffer with ailments such as back
pain and incontinence often associated with poor pressure
management within the core.*

*TAKE BREAKS FROM THE SHOULDER BLADES OFF THE
FLOOR POSITION AS NEEDED. You can perform this test in
several stages (performing several "mini-lifts") as you work
your way down the midline (the linea alba). Taking breaks will
help you to avoid sustained intra-abdominal pressure in this
potentially weakened area.*

If you have an unclosed DR, you have special needs when it comes to core
fitness and caring for your abdominal muscles. This is true if you're four
months (or 14 years) postpartum. But there's good news! With proper
care of your abdomen and appropriate inner core strengthening, the gap
should lessen and the integrity of the linea alba will increase over time.
I encourage you to seek individualized advice from a post-natal fitness
specialist or a women's health physical therapist, but in the meantime,
these tips will help:

- "Zip up" (engage your core muscles from your pelvic floor on up
  through your low abs) when lifting/pushing/pulling.

- Get out of bed without "jack-knifing." In other words, don't sit
  bolt upright! Roll to your side first, and then push yourself up to

a seated position.

- Always, always, always, "exhale on exertion."

- Sit less and move more. Too much sitting leads to tight hip flexors, which can pull your posture out of alignment, exaggerating the lumbar curve and making your tummy protrude.

- Practice good posture. As discussed in the previous chapter, this also helps with back pain, bladder health, and bone health.

- Use core breathing as a great way to build inner core strength.

- Eat plenty of gelatin and bone broth to provide your body the collagen it needs to help heal the DR. Learn more about these superfoods in Chapter 14.

- Eat unprocessed, "clean" foods to support your body's healing processes in general. We'll discuss clean eating in Chapter 14.

The most important thing to remember is that you can make the separation worse by doing the wrong exercises. Many new mothers are anxious to return to their pre-baby body and embark on an intense abdominal program including crunches, sit-ups, and other exercises that focus on trunk flexion. Crunches and sit-ups have their place in the world of core strengthening, but they should be avoided for women with DR. Until you've healed, crunches can make your diastasis larger.

You should also be cautious with planks and exercises that are done on your hands and knees. These exercises are not completely off-limits, but doing too many of them – and doing them without properly engaging the deep abdominal muscles – can be an issue due to the weight of the viscera (abdominal organs) pushing against the weak abdominal wall.

The exercises in the Inner Core Energizer routine are – for the most part – safe for women with DR; however, there are a few exercises that may need to be modified. I have made notes for these modifications, so if you are healing from DR, please watch for them and follow the instructions carefully!

If you have specific questions about healing from DR, MuTu® System for postpartum women gets rave reviews (www.mutusystem.com). I can also recommend physical therapist Marianne Ryan's new book, *Baby Bod*, for learning how to activate your deep core muscles safely and effectively. If you're a health or fitness professional and want to learn more about serving your postnatal clients using holistic DR healing and C-section recovery methods, check out Burrell Education (www.burrelleducation.com). See the Resources section for more information.

CHILDBIRTH AND THE PELVIC FLOOR

Childbirth itself puts the pelvic floor muscles at risk. Difficult deliveries can damage the pelvic floor muscles due to tearing, which can be extreme enough to lacerate the pelvic floor muscles themselves. In severe situations (third and fourth degree lacerations), the tears can extend all the way to – and even through – the anus. This can lead to fecal incontinence and/or difficulty controlling gas, and can also contribute to painful sex.

Prolonged pressure on nerves in the pelvic region is another risk women undergo during labor. In most cases, prolonged pressure on the nerves causes only temporary dysfunction, but longstanding nerve damage can occur in severe cases. Extended pushing phases can contribute to pelvic organ prolapse, which is when the pelvic organs (specifically the bladder, uterus, and/or rectum) "hang a little low" and press into the vaginal wall, or – as in the case of uterine prolapse – slip down into (and may protrude out of) the vagina. Pelvic organ prolapse is extremely common, with reports of it being experienced – to some degree – by up to 50% of parous women (women who have given birth).[19]

Pelvic floor risk is not limited to women who deliver babies vaginally; even women who have C-sections can have problems related to pelvic floor muscle weakness and overstretching due to nine (plus) months of downward pressure on the pelvic floor muscles during pregnancy, and the possibility of hours of pushing prior to surgery (if the C-section was unplanned). Regardless of mode of delivery, maintaining strong and flexible pelvic floor muscles should be an important part of **every woman's** prenatal and postpartum plans.

Currently pregnant? For a free pregnancy exercise tutorial designed by women's health physical therapist Tasha Mulligan, go to *www.hab-it.com/videos-preg.html*.

PELVIC ORGAN PROLAPSE

Pelvic organ prolapse – when one or more of the pelvic organs descend or slip out of place – is not related to pregnancy alone. In my practice as a physical therapist I worked with multiple nulliparous (never borne offspring) women who experienced problems related to pelvic floor and core weakness. One of my nulliparous patients was a professional landscaper who had engaged in a long and successful career. Externally, she looked like she was in great shape, but when I completed an internal pelvic floor muscle examination I found that her pelvic floor was weak and uncoordinated and that she was suffering from significant uterine prolapse. Years of lifting heavy loads with improper body mechanics had pushed her uterus downward and had taken a toll on her pelvic floor muscles.

Prolapse presents differently in different women. Some are completely asymptomatic, whereas others report discomfort during sex, a feeling of weakness "down below," aching pelvic discomfort or back pain that gets worse as the day goes on, and/or sensations likened to a golf ball in their vagina, or like a tampon that's stuck in the wrong place.

What can you do to prevent prolapse? First and foremost, recall the importance of posture (discussed in the previous chapter). To prevent prolapse or the progression of prolapse, you have to be sure that your posture and alignment are spot-on. Repeatedly standing or sitting with poor posture puts excessive pressure on your abdominal and pelvic organs and strains your muscles and connective tissues.

"Is there anything else I can do?"

Toilet habits are important to consider when it comes to preventing prolapse, or preventing progression of prolapse that has already begun. Make sure you are staying regular and that you don't have to strain to have a bowel movement. Keep your stools soft and easy to pass by eating a diet rich in liquids from water and soups, and high in fiber, primarily from veggies, fruits, and moderate amounts of nuts and seeds. Chia seeds are a great example. Pop online and search for chia recipes – you might be surprised at how popular this high-fiber ingredient has become.

Another way to prevent straining during a bowel movement is to place your feet on a stepstool or even two yoga blocks (one on either side of the toilet) so that your knees are above your hips when having a bowel movement. If you keep your spine straight, this recreates a squatting position, which is the position from which our bodies were designed to eliminate.

Furthermore, don't push to pee. This is a common habit, especially amongst time-stressed mothers and workers whose clients depend on them all day long, such as nurses and teachers. When people are clamoring for your attention, and truly need you to be there for them, it can be difficult to spare even thirty seconds to urinate in a relaxed fashion. But this is essential for the health of your pelvic floor muscles and to prevent prolapse. You MUST allow yourself 30-60 seconds to fully empty your bladder!

Two negative things can happen when you rush the toileting process. First, you probably aren't allowing all of the urine to release. This leads to incomplete bladder evacuation and the feeling that you "always have to go." Second, if you're trying to release all of your urine, but doing so in a hurry, you're probably straining. As described above, when you strain (bear down) to urinate more quickly, or to make sure you've emptied your bladder all the way, it puts a tremendous amount of pressure on the pelvic organs and the pelvic floor. **Let things flow out naturally!** When you're on the toilet, don't worry about getting the deed done quickly. Take your time. If you feel like your bladder doesn't fully empty without a little "push" from you, then try this: rather than pushing, rock your pelvis back and forth slowly while still seated on the toilet. This tips your bladder back and forth and uses gravity to help siphon out every last drop.

Speaking of being seated on the toilet, do not "hover." When I was in clinical practice, I was shocked by the number of women with bladder control issues who admitted to "hovering" above the toilet seat to urinate. I encouraged all of my patients who "hovered" (rather than sitting fully on the toilet) to stop this habit immediately! If sanitation is a concern, use a toilet seat liner. If a liner is unavailable, then line the toilet seat with toilet paper...or just take a risk and sit down on the seat! A person's bottom and upper thighs, which are covered most of the day, are usually much cleaner than a person's hands, and we tend to have no qualms about social situations that require a handshake.

So please, sit and relax when you need to pee.

The problem with "hovering" above the toilet seat while urinating is that it causes the muscles of your pelvic floor and pelvic girdle (i.e. your hip rotators, buttocks, back, and abs) to be extremely tense. This muscular tension makes it difficult for urine to flow easily, often requiring you to bear down slightly to initiate urination. You may also find yourself pushing to make the urine flow out faster, because it's hard work hovering above the toilet! Your thighs are burning, and you're thinking, "Let's just hurry this along!" But as you now know, frequent pushing or bearing down to urinate can contribute to pelvic organ prolapse.

Even if you don't push to urinate when "hovering," due to the tension in the pelvic floor and core muscles you may not fully empty your bladder. This can lead to incomplete evacuation of the bladder, which may ultimately cause increased frequency and urgency of urination, or in extreme cases, can increase your risk of developing urinary tract infections.[20]

More on prolapse prevention...

Body mechanics are key. Body mechanics, or the way you use your body to complete your daily physical activities, are extremely important to consider when it comes to preventing prolapse (or preventing the progression of prolapse that has already begun). **Remember to exhale on exertion, and this simple phrase: "Seal it off."** Repetitively lifting babies (and then toddlers, and then preschoolers), weight lifting, and heavy manual labor are fantastic natural activities and completely safe for women to do when using proper body mechanics; however, women have special needs that are rarely taught and must be considered. When lifting heavy things, you need to exhale as you lift and remember to "zip up" your inner core. Start by "sealing off" the pelvic floor. This will protect your back and will prevent issues such as pelvic organ prolapse.

Here's a visualization that will help you really understand the importance of sealing off the pelvic floor muscles prior to lifting something heavy: Think of a full toothpaste tube that's NOT capped. When you put downward pressure on the toothpaste tube by squeezing from the top, what happens to the toothpaste? It splurts out.

This is an excellent – if not dramatic – parallel to what can happen to the pelvic organs when downward pressure is applied (via heavy lifting) and the pelvic floor muscles are either weak, not functioning properly, or not properly engaged.

Imagine that while weight lifting you do a "clean and jerk" lift with weak and/or un-engaged pelvic floor and core muscles. You squat down and then jerk the barbell up – which causes an incredible amount of downward force on the pelvic floor – and...splat. Either an accident will occur (bladder control issues are reported to be fairly common among female CrossFit® athletes), or over time, you'll develop an increased risk for pelvic organ prolapse.

Let's talk about crunches and sit-ups, two classic abdominal strengthening exercises. Returning to the visual of the uncapped toothpaste tube, now imagine bending it in the middle. What happens to the toothpaste? Again, it splurts out. This is analogous to an abdominal crunch (or any other core exercise that involves trunk flexion) with weak and/or un-engaged pelvic floor and core muscles. You bend at the waist to "crunch" and...splat. Repeated downward pressure on your pelvic organs without support from below (from the pelvic floor) puts you at significant risk for developing pelvic organ prolapse.

So the moral of the story – "seal off" your pelvic floor and "zip up" your core when lifting heavy things and doing abdominal exercises. Most importantly, do your best to keep your pelvic floor and core muscles strong and supple. Walk! Squat whenever you can! Move more! Do exercises such as those found in this book! Make love on a regular basis! You'll look better, feel better, and help prevent prolapse, which can be an uncomfortable and disheartening condition.

IMPORTANT NOTE: You don't need to "seal off" and "zip up" all day long... No, no, no. Conscious, active "zipping" is only required when you are:

- Doing something strenuous or moderately strenuous, such as lifting, bending, pushing, or pulling (some examples: moving a box, lifting your dog, vacuuming).

- Doing focused core strengthening exercises or weight lifting/ resistance training.

- Doing activities that require extra stability, balance, and control (such as standing on a ladder and reaching out to paint something).

- Doing things that might be jarring to the pelvic floor such as jumping, running, etc.

At other times – during normal, non-rigorous activities of daily living – don't worry about "sealing off" or "zipping." Simply use good posture and relax the core. Your core muscles are always firing – always slightly on – throughout the day. If they weren't on, you wouldn't be able to stand up. Zipping makes them "extra on," and you do NOT want to overly tax your muscles by zipping up the core all day long. Too much zipping can create excess muscle tension and ultimately pain and dysfunction.

"I've heard about pessaries. Are they a good option?"

A pessary is a device that can be inserted into the vagina in order to provide support of prolapsed pelvic organs. Pessaries can be a great solution for some women, and an alternative to more invasive measures such as surgical repair of the prolapse. My personal approach is to encourage clients to exhaust all conservative treatment options such as core and pelvic floor strengthening, posture training, toileting habits, body mechanics, and even a trial of pessary use, BEFORE resorting to surgery. That being said, when prolapse is too far advanced and begins to cause pain or interfere with a person's daily life, surgical intervention may be necessary. This is a conversation to have with a gynecologist or urogynecologist.

INCONTINENCE

Incontinence (bladder leakage) is a common occurrence among women of all ages and stages; even young women are not exempt. I have worked with several women in their late teens and early twenties who were heavily involved in athletics and experienced uncontrollable urinary leakage. One of my younger patients loved dodge ball which, when played competitively as an adult, is incredibly intense! The sport involves high impact, fast-paced activities such as running, jumping, throwing, catching, and (of course) **dodging**. Although my patient was athletic and strong, her inner core muscles were not as fit as they needed to be in order to prevent leakage during competitive games.

Fun Tidbit: Are you a runner? The jarring effects of pavement pounding and other high impact exercises can cause you to reach (and exceed) your "continence threshold" more quickly than lower impact fitness activities. The continence threshold corresponds to the amount of force and the length of time with which the pelvic floor muscles can withstand the effects of repetitive impact. This threshold is reached must faster if the pelvic floor muscles have not been sufficiently prepared for high impact activities.

Now, this isn't to say that you should "zip up" or hold a kegel throughout your twenty-mile run in order to prevent prolapse and bladder leakage... Just be sure that your baseline level of core and pelvic floor strength is sufficient.

Runners – and I know this, because I once identified primarily as a runner – can be guilty of focusing SO MUCH on their endurance training that they neglect cross-training and doing other activities that strengthen their core. Try adding a Pilates class, a yoga class that focuses on core strength and control, or bellydance lessons to your running program. If you have determined that kegels are an appropriate exercise for you, then do 5-10 "endurance" kegels daily. And be sure to squat regularly! The Inner Core Energizer routine in Chapter 13 is a great place to start.

Incontinence is typically divided into three primary types: stress, urge, and mixed. Although a sudden onset of loss of bladder control is a concern that should be discussed immediately with your doctor, most cases of incontinence are quite treatable using simple techniques such as pelvic floor and core strengthening, and bladder retraining.

Stress incontinence is bladder leakage (even just a small amount) with physical stressors, such as running, jumping, coughing, laughing, or sneezing. All of these activities put significant downward pressure on your bladder and pelvic floor muscles, and can lead to an accident if you have pelvic floor dysfunction.

If you have stress incontinence, remember the pelvic brace technique that was described in Chapter 8. In short, you must consciously contract your pelvic floor muscles **prior to** activities that create an increase in intra-abdominal pressure, such as lifting, coughing, and blowing your nose. This will help "seal off" the urethra and prevent bladder leakage.

Urge incontinence, often referred to as "overactive bladder," is bladder leakage (even just a small amount) associated with a feeling of urinary urgency. If you've ever thought, *"I've gotta go... RIGHT NOW!"* and not made it to the bathroom on time, then you have experienced urge incontinence. It can also play out as bladder leakage when unbuttoning your pants to use the toilet, a sudden urge (and leakage) when walking by running water, or a sensation of having to urinate several times during the night, and frequently – sometimes ridiculously so – during the day, as well.

Urge incontinence is often successfully treated with bladder retraining techniques (best done under the supervision of a women's health physical therapist or other qualified medical practitioner). Bladder retraining gradually trains your body – and mind – to use the restroom less frequently, often utilizing a "bladder diary" to keep track of when you're urinating, how much you're urinating (volume-wise), and how much fluid you're consuming.

Mixed incontinence is a combination of stress and urge incontinence. As indicated above, a significant contributor to both urge and mixed incontinence is bladder hypersensitivity. If you never fully empty your bladder due to rushing or "hovering" over the toilet seat – or if you find yourself running to the bathroom the minute you feel the first sensation that you need to pee – you may develop a highly sensitive bladder. Bladder retraining can help, as can limiting your intake of caffeine and alcohol, losing weight if you are overweight, and calming your nervous system by deeply breathing when you feel an urge to urinate.

If you suffer from any type of incontinence, please do not be ashamed. Don't keep it to yourself; there is help! A women's health physical therapist can help determine a treatment plan based on your specific needs.

HYSTERECTOMY

A hysterectomy is the surgical removal of the uterus (womb). Accompanying organs may or may not be removed at the same time. In a "partial" or supracervical hysterectomy, the upper part of the uterus is removed, leaving the cervix intact. In a complete or "total" hysterectomy, both the uterus and the cervix are removed. In a hysterectomy with bilateral salpingo-oophorectomy (try saying that 5 times fast!), the uterus, cervix, fallopian tubes, and ovaries are removed. A "radical" hysterectomy is an extensive surgical procedure in which the uterus, cervix, ovaries, fallopian tubes, upper vagina, and lymph nodes are removed.

Hysterectomies are performed to treat conditions such as fibroids, heavy menstrual bleeding, endometriosis (when uterine tissue grows outside of the lining of the uterus), adenomyosis (when endometrial tissue grows into the muscle wall of the uterus), uterine prolapse, and cancer. In the case of prolapse, hysterectomies should be reserved for women for whom more conservative treatment options have not worked.

There are three primary approaches for hysterectomy surgery: abdominal, vaginal, and laparoscopic. Although these approaches are very different, all three require invasion of the tissues in the abdominal and pelvic regions.

A hysterectomy is a major surgery, and as with ANY major surgery there are risks involved. These risks include post-surgical infection, excessive bleeding, and/or complications associated with anesthesia. More specific to hysterectomy, post-surgical complications may also include urinary complaints, a possible decrease in sexual responsiveness if the cervix is removed, a decrease in production of sex hormones depending on which structures are removed, and an increased risk of vaginal vault prolapse. Vaginal vault prolapse can occur when the top of the vagina drops down as a result of a reduction in support structures (i.e. the uterus, fallopian tubes, and cervix).

Patients who undergo a hysterectomy must understand that they will not be able to conceive after the surgery, and that there may be some hormonal changes that can force early menopause or require hormone replacement therapy. **The decision to have a hysterectomy is complex and often very emotional, and something that should be thoroughly considered and discussed with your healthcare provider. Seek a second opinion if your intuition makes you wonder whether or not it is absolutely necessary in your case.**

Based on your condition, there are questions you might want to ask your doctor or surgeon. It's a good idea to bring your questions in writing, and possibly bring a support person along with you, as well. Some questions you might consider asking include:

- Are there any other procedures or treatments I can try first, before a hysterectomy?

- Will my condition continue to get worse without surgery, or not?

- Will my ovaries or other reproductive organs (other than my uterus) be removed during the procedure? If so, what are the implications?

- Will my cervix be removed during the surgery? What are the pros and cons of removing the cervix versus leaving it intact?

- Will the surgery you are recommending cause menopause? If so, what are your recommendations?

- Will you be using an abdominal, vaginal, or laparoscopic technique? What are the pros and cons of each technique?

- What are the chances my symptoms could reoccur after surgery?

- How many procedures have you performed in the last 12 months of this type?

- What is the recovery time? When can I resume my normal activities including work, sex, and physical activities?

- May I talk to one of your patients who has had the same type of hysterectomy you are recommending for me?[21]

Be sure you're comfortable with your surgeon prior to scheduling surgery. You want to feel supported by your surgeon, and fully confident in their skills as well as their ability (and willingness) to answer your questions openly and honestly. Do you leave their office feeling reassured and uplifted? Do you feel heard? Do you feel like you're in good hands? If not, ask around and seek a different provider. Often, the best referrals are from other patients or someone who knows the practitioner personally, such as a nurse who has worked with local surgeons and can provide a good recommendation.

The power of word of mouth – of being in partnership with your healthcare provider, and of women talking to women – is strong.

One of my clients, Kristen, underwent a sling procedure and partial hysterectomy to treat incontinence, cystocele (bladder prolapse), and rectocele (prolapse of the rectum). Kristen had minimal information going into surgery, was not prompted to attempt any form of conservative treatment prior to surgery, and didn't consider seeking a second opinion. She states:

"If I had known about the chance of early onset menopause and the more rapid aging of my vagina BEFORE I'd had my hysterectomy, I probably wouldn't

have had the surgery, or would have at least delayed it. **I wish that we, as a culture, would speak more openly about these issues that affect so many of us as we age.** *If my older friends had talked about things like incontinence, prolapse, and going through menopause more openly, it would have been easier to make an informed decision about my own surgery... My own health!"*

Starting these types of conversations is one of the driving forces behind this book. I don't have all the answers, and neither will your friends or the Internet or even your doctor. But the more we talk and share stories, personal experiences, research, and information, the more we open the door for all of us to make fully informed decisions.

> **Fun Tidbit:** Phantom womb sensations. If you've had a hysterectomy, it's still likely that you can sense your womb energy as described in the section titled "Womb Power" (Chapter 5). Try the exercise for tapping into your creative center, which is still present, albeit changed. Your womb was with you for years, and left an imprint – physical, emotional, and energetic. Place your hands on your lower abdomen, over the place where your uterus was. Feel into the feminine energy that remains.

BACK PAIN

Back pain is one of the most common patient complaints in the United States. Low back pain affects 5.6 percent of American adults each day, with 18 percent reporting back pain in the previous month.[22] Relapses are common and the pain can be debilitating, causing many sufferers to seek medication and often requiring time off work to recuperate. Between healthcare costs and lost labor, mechanical back pain costs Americans billions of dollars each year.

Mechanical back pain refers to pain that is caused by abnormal stress and strain on the muscles of the vertebral column. It is usually the cumulative result of years of bad habits such as poor posture, a sedentary lifestyle, weakness of the core muscles, and improper body mechanics when lifting, bending, and pushing.

Approximately two thirds of adults are affected by mechanical low back pain at some point in their lives; onset of pain usually occurs at some point between 30-50 years of age.[23] It is also a common complaint during and after pregnancy due to the postural and musculoskeletal changes that occur as the uterus and abdomen enlarge.

Unfortunately, most adult Americans are destined for back pain unless they make a concerted effort to alter (and improve) their postural habits, use proper body mechanics, and increase core strength. **Moving your body in all directions and regularly participating in a fitness program such as the Inner Core Energizer is the best prevention (and treatment) for mechanical back pain.** In short: MOVE MORE.

"But when my back hurts, I don't want to move!"

I completely understand, and agree that when you're in pain, you should take it easy to avoid aggravating your symptoms. However, if you take the prescription of "rest" to the extreme and simply STOP moving, you will experience stiffness and decreased circulation to the affected joints, muscles, and nerves. Ultimately, this causes even more pain and dysfunction. It's a fine line, and definitely one that should be explored with a licensed physical therapist or other qualified healthcare practitioner. But please take this message to heart: Motion is lotion, and – in the long run – movement makes everything better. Gentle, regular movement helps the body function optimally and has numerous preventative health benefits.

Want an easy way to prevent back pain (and possibly even treat mild cases of pain)? Try the "30-30 Rule." **It's simple: Whatever you've been doing for the last 30 minutes, spend 30 seconds doing the OPPOSITE.**

For example, if you realize that you've been sitting at your computer with your head jutted forward and your shoulders rounded as you browse the Internet or update social media, STOP! Close your eyes, pull your chin back toward your neck (i.e. give yourself a "double chin" in order to stretch the muscles at the base of your skull and behind your neck), and roll your shoulders back and down. Clasp your hands behind your back to really open your chest.

If your low back is bothering you, take 30 seconds to stand up and do a supported back bend (place your hands on your hips for support as you extend your spine and arch your back). A quick side-bend or two, or a couple of hip circles, are also nice options.

And if you realize that you haven't taken a deep, relaxing breath in the last 30 minutes (often we breathe so shallowly that our lungs rarely get a chance to fully expand), then take 30 seconds to do so now. Every muscle in your body will thank you.

EXERCISE – The 30-30 Rule:

Stop what you're doing, right now. Take 30 seconds to move your body and/or stretch in the opposite direction.

SCIATICA

Many women have experienced sciatica, a burning pain that shoots from the low back or buttocks down to the calf – or even all the way down to the foot – on one or both sides of the body. This neuro-musculo-skeletal condition is best treated by a physical therapist or other qualified healthcare provider, but you can get a head start on treatment by understanding the basics of sciatica.

The main "gist" is that a large nerve – the sciatic nerve, the longest nerve in the human body – becomes irritated and inflamed and sends searing pain along its path (down the leg, from the sacrum to the foot). One reason the sciatic nerve can become irritated is compression: it travels between, over, and through the deep hip and gluteal muscles. If any of these muscles are tight or excessively tense, they can compress the sciatic nerve, contributing to pain. This is a great reason to keep your hip muscles flexible, strong, and supple by regularly walking, moving, stretching, changing positions, and doing exercises such as those found in the Inner Core Energizer.

Another reason the sciatic nerve can become irritated is poor posture and improper alignment. When your pelvis is off-kilter, the muscles that surround the joints in the spine, pelvis, and hips are also off-kilter. Again, the sciatic nerve travels through this very complex region of muscles, joints, and connective tissue, so any type of bony misalignment (and the resulting "angry" muscles that will occur) can compromise the sciatic nerve and cause sciatica. This is one reason sciatica is extremely common during pregnancy – since pregnancy contributes to postural changes, sciatica often crops up.

In any case, if you begin to experience muscle weakness, numbness or tingling, you need to seek medical attention immediately.

NECK PAIN, TENSION, AND HEADACHES

Do you carry tension in your shoulders? Many women do, which can result in neck pain, mid-back and upper-back pain, and even headaches.

A top contributor to upper body tension and pain includes improper ergonomics at work and holding single positions for too long. Be sure your workstation is appropriately fitted for your body. Do you jut your head forward throughout the day in order to see your computer screen? Do you type on a keyboard that's too high or too low and causes your shoulders to hitch up or round forward? When you're at home, do you prepare food on a counter that's too high or too low? Do you nurse your baby with rounded shoulders and a forward head? Change your work environment to fit your body, and change positions often to prevent tension from accumulating. Remember the 30-30 Rule!

Another contributor to neck pain and headaches is shallow, high-in-your-chest breathing, which is common when you're under stress. We'll be talking more about breathing and relaxation in Chapter 11. It's amazing how quickly tension headaches can be relieved when you learn how to breathe properly.

You might be sensing some common themes! When it comes to musculoskeletal conditions, finding and maintaining proper posture, regularly moving your body, and relaxation and stress management techniques are essential. Massage, chiropractic care, and acupuncture may also be helpful. The key point to remember is this: don't blow off caring for yourself! Make the necessary lifestyle changes (or seek treatment) before the condition gets so severe that it interferes with daily life. Take care of yourself now so you can be the light later.

> **"The wound is the place where the Light enters you."**
> **–Rumi**

WEIGHT GAIN

As any female can attest, it gets harder to shake off extra pounds as you age. On a physical level, excess weight is directly correlated with an increase in urinary incontinence.[24] Excess abdominal fat in particular is associated with insulin resistance, chronic systemic inflammation, and even increased risk of certain cancers.[25] On an emotional and spiritual level, excess weight can lead to struggles – sometimes for life – with body image, self-love, and self-acceptance.

Genetics, lifestyle, hormones, and metabolism play leading roles in your weight and the relative ease or difficulty with which you lose it. But there's another, lesser-known reason for weight gain (and retention). We are sensory beings, and as a society – especially as women – we have been taught that it's not okay to experience pleasure with eating, and that if we have, we've violated certain rules such as, "You should only eat to live," that "If you eat that you're going to get fat," and that you "should" look a certain way. These built-in false beliefs often lead to binge eating, emotional eating, compulsive eating, closet eating (eating in secret), and feeling addicted to food.

Food can be used as a drug, and it can be nearly as destructive when used in this way! After the initial pleasure, food "users" eat more to get another "hit." But it just doesn't work… "After a certain point, the pleasure is gone and it just becomes a way of numbing out," says Dr. Joy Jacobs, a clinical psychologist, coach, and author specializing in issues related to eating, weight management, and body image.[26] The first thing

Dr. Jacobs does to help her clients lose weight is to make them commit to stop dieting, because as she says, traditional (usually restrictive) diets result in a feeling of deprivation that can build up over time, leading to compensatory over-eating and ultimately, the "yo-yo" effect.

The take home message – weight loss is much more complex than eating fewer calories and exercising more. Eating nutrient-dense, high quality foods, moderating your food intake (not too much, but also not too little), getting enough sleep, managing your stress, **loving and accepting** yourself, and moving regularly are the safest ways to effectively lose weight and keep it off. It is absolutely essential to learn how to ENJOY clean eating and moving every day in order to keep your metabolism stoked and your body healthy as you age.

BLOATING AND CONSTIPATION

Have you ever had one of those days when you open the closet, and nothing feels right? Do you ever spend 45 minutes searching through your clothes, just trying to find an outfit that will hide your bloated belly? You're not alone. Bloating is a common symptom among women of all ages, and it can wreak havoc on your body image and certainly your comfort level.

It is important to note that persistent bloating is a warning sign for polycystic ovarian syndrome (PCOS), endometriosis, and certain types of cancers such as ovarian cancer. However, on a less pathological (but still problematic) level, bloating can also be a symptom of imbalanced gut flora, food intolerance(s), and/or too much fermentation in the digestive tract…usually a constipated, plugged-up digestive tract.

Everybody poops. Make sure you do, too!

Did you know that Americans spend more than $700 million on laxatives each year?[27] Getting Americans to poop is a booming industry! If you struggle with constipation, there are plenty of natural (laxative-free) treatment options.

As Nadya Andreeva, author of *Happy Belly*, states, "Feeling feminine, sexy, playful, and flirty is almost impossible when we feel bad about our own body. A distended stomach, cramps, feeling stuck down there from carrying around several days of waste. . . is anything but sexy. It kills the desire for intimacy!" [28]

Before figuring out my own personal dietary needs, I had struggled with constipation for years. I thought I was alone before starting my work as a women's health physical therapist. Certainly, many of my patients struggled with diarrhea and the feeling that food "moved right through them," but more often than not, I heard about constipation. I was astounded by the number of clients and friends who thought nothing of the fact that they might only have one bowel movement per week. Ladies, there are a lot of wacky things that are normal...but pooping once per week is not normal, and it's not okay!

As stated in Dr. Pratima Raichur's Ayurvedic skin care guide *Absolute Beauty*, "The dietary principles for staying young and beautiful are universal: keep the colon clean and the digestion strong."[29] How can this be accomplished in today's fast food, fast-paced, highly toxic world? Simply aim for a great bowel movement every day.

What does a great bowel movement look like? Take a look at the Bristol Stool Chart (searchable online) and shoot for a 3-5. Most sources say 3-4 is best, others have referenced 4-5 as ideal... I think that 3, 4, and 5 are all great as long as the bowel movements are happening regularly and easily, without having to strain.

Always remember the ultimate goal, which is to keep your "pipes" running smoothly in order to release the gunk and junk that can prematurely age your body.

Not pooping every day? Try these tips:

- Avoid foods that are inflammatory; they clog you up and weigh you down. These include: refined sugar, refined white flour, artificial sweeteners, chemically fed, chemically treated, genetically altered or irradiated foods, artificial coloring, "no fat" foods made with fat substitutes (usually extra sugar), deep fried fast foods and other foods cooked in reused oils, and any product with trans fats (often found in margarine sticks, pre-made frostings, boxed cake and biscuit mixes, store-bought cookies and cookie dough, restaurant shakes and creamy drinks, frozen TV dinners, and certain brands of canned chili and packaged pudding). Read labels and check ingredients. A good rule of thumb is if you can't pronounce it, don't buy it.

• Allow your previous meal to digest before eating your next meal or snack. **Try to wait at least three hours between meals to avoid a backlog of undigested food in your system.**

• **Chew well and don't talk while chewing.** Digestion actually begins in the mouth, with your salivary enzymes, so give your body a chance to start the digestion process off right by chewing fully! If you're eating with others, put down your fork between bites and let the flavor and the experience of food be your only focus.

• **Be careful with your fiber.** Some women thrive on a diet rich in whole grains, legumes, and pulses (i.e. brown rice, beans, and lentils). For other women, this type of diet would chain them to the toilet with diarrhea or loose stools. For still others, it would cause gas, bloating, and constipation.

Although it is important to get sufficient fiber in your diet (and many modern diets do NOT include enough fiber), some individuals consume more than their bodies can handle. If you are consciously eating sufficient fiber (25-35 grams/day) but are still constipated, you might need to drink more water to help flush the fiber through, or you might actually need to decrease dietary fiber, at least for a time, and increase healthy fats and nourishing liquids such as bone broth. This can help ease the passage of solids through the gut, and can also help heal the gut lining if there is any inflammation present.

This is a slight tangent, but it's an important consideration for women, specifically: Eating too much fiber may actually decrease fertility in some women due to decreased hormone concentrations (estradiol, progesterone, LH, and FSH) and a higher likelihood of anovulation. In a 2009 study of 250 women aged 18–44, fruit fiber had the strongest association with decreased concentrations of estradiol, followed by grain fiber.[30] It is unclear exactly "how much is too much," but to be on the safe side, if you're interested in getting pregnant, you might want to err on the side of caution and stick to the lower end of the recommended range (don't go beyond 25 grams of fiber per day).

- Avoid eating fruit **after a meal**. This habit is gas-forming and leads to bloating. Consider this your cue to "eat dessert first!"

- **Stay hydrated.** Start your day with a large glass of lukewarm water. Try adding some lemon juice and a pinch of cayenne pepper to rev metabolism and warm your body from the inside out. Hydration requirements vary depending on your individual body type and activity level, but as a general rule, listen to your body and heed the signal of thirst. If you like numbers, aim for 50-60 ounces of water throughout each day and increase (or decrease) from there.

- **Speaking of fluids, don't drink anything cold while eating.** Too much cold (from fluids or food) can inhibit digestion. This is based on an Ayurvedic principle, which states that an abundance of cold will squelch your digestive fire, and it is confirmed by my own personal experience.

- Another Ayurvedic remedy to help soothe a stubbornly slow OR an overly active digestive tract is to **chew on fennel seeds or sip a hot fennel tea**. A traditional dose of fennel tea is about two to three cups daily. If you're at a restaurant or don't have fennel seeds, opt for ginger or mint teas, which are also soothing to the digestive tract.

- **Move your body!** Movement increases blood flow throughout the body and helps aid peristalsis (the natural movement of the gut that helps propel food through your GI tract). Walking, hip circles, twists (i.e. upper body twists, or twisting stretches such as those found in certain yoga practices), and jumping on a mini trampoline all **help to increase blood circulation, stimulate lymphatic flow, and to release gas**. I love starting my day with 50 hip circles in each direction. If I'm constipated, I'll go for a 30-minute walk. Like magic, the toilet beckons the minute I return home.

- Speaking of peristalsis, **gentle abdominal massage** can help cultivate and assist your gut's natural peristaltic action. Gently massage your abdomen in a clockwise direction for 10-15 minutes every day. The aim is to follow the path that food and waste travel when moving through your large intestine. To do it, lie down comfortably, and use gentle pressure with the tips of your fingers (from one or both hands) to massage in gentle, circular motions up the path of the ascending colon, which is on the right side of your abdomen. Then gently massage over the transverse colon (located in the top of the abdomen just below your ribs) traveling from the right side to the left. Finally, massage down the path of the descending colon, which is on the left side of your abdomen. NOTE: This type of massage is contraindicated for people with a bowel obstruction or abdominal growth, or for those with inflammatory bowel disease, Crohn's disease, or ulcerative colitis. Talk to your healthcare provider if you have additional questions or concerns about your specific health condition.

- **Prioritize adequate unstructured, unhurried time in the morning.** This is the ideal time for elimination since your organs have been naturally detoxifying your body overnight, but you need to be relaxed in order to fully release. If you hit the ground running when the alarm rings and then rush out the door, you are unlikely to have a full (and satisfactory) bowel movement.

- As described in the section on prolapse, take your time so that you can fully evacuate your bowels and **consider placing your feet on a step stool** or specifically designed toilet stool to mimic a squatting position. This helps prevent straining and can lead to an easier, faster elimination and less risk for pelvic organ prolapse from repetitive straining.

- **Supplement with seeds.** Try incorporating 1 Tablespoon of ground flaxseeds or 1 Tablespoon of chia seeds into your diet each day. Sprinkle ground flaxseeds on salads, veggies, or blend into smoothies. Incorporate chia into smoothies (beware – chia thickens any liquid!), gluten-free oatmeal, or grain-free porridge.

- **Inoculate your gut with good bacteria.** Purchase a broad-spectrum probiotic supplement. Start with a low dose (you can even break the capsule in half and sprinkle it into your food or beverage) and work your way up to the recommended dosage. Everyone reacts differently to probiotics, and individuals with Small Intestinal Bacterial Overgrowth (SIBO) or other chronic gut conditions may have special needs when it comes to probiotic use. If you have any questions or concerns, or have any type of untoward reaction after using a probiotic, please consult with a naturopathic doctor or functional medicine practitioner for a personalized plan.

- **Consider magnesium supplementation.** Magnesium deficiency is common, with symptoms ranging from constipation to anxiety, muscle cramps, and insomnia. I love using "Natural Calm" (made by the brand Natural Vitality) magnesium citrate. I take a dose before bed; it not only helps me sleep well, it also keeps me regular. Start with a low dose and work up to the recommended dosage if needed. I find that just 1 teaspoon per day is perfect for me. Again, if you have any questions or concerns, please consult with a naturopathic doctor or functional medicine practitioner.

The above recommendations can be used on a daily basis. Below are tips you can use if you experience periodic bouts of constipation (not for daily use). Questions or concerns? Consult with your naturopathic doctor or functional medicine practitioner.

- **VITAMIN C SUPPLEMENTATION:** Try taking 1000-2000 mg of buffered ascorbic acid (Vitamin C) powder or capsules if you need to loosen your stools quickly. This may also help with detoxification and inflammation. Look for a brand that also contains bioflavonoids for maximum absorption.

- **LAST DITCH EFFORT:** Use a gentle herbal laxative as directed. This should be a short-term "fix" rather than a regular part of your routine.

STRESS

Stress is rampant in our society and women are significantly impacted by it. Lack of sleep, too many commitments, and over-working take a toll on our minds and bodies, dimming our radiance and robbing us of our mojo.

From painful periods to sleepless nights to weight gain to skin issues, we all react to stress differently, but the common denominator is the same – too much stress can cause hormonal imbalance and/or systemic inflammation, both of which are the underlying cause of hundreds of devastating and debilitating chronic illnesses.

The following bottle analogy symbolizes the cumulative impact of stress over time. Imagine holding an empty soda bottle, or even a baby bottle, with your arm straight out in front of you. For the first minute or two, the bottle weighs next-to-nothing. But imagine that you have to keep holding the bottle straight out in front of you for an hour, or eight hours...or a month...or a year. Your body would be screaming!

Like a bottle, our stressors can initially appear harmless (or weightless), but when carried day in and day out, they add up and weigh you down.

My "canary in a coal mine" (my warning sign that I'm over-stressed) is a small patch of psoriasis on my right knee. Interestingly, the right side of the body correlates with masculine or "doing" energy, which tends to be my dominant energy. When I'm over-done (over-worked, over-exercised, over-worried), my psoriasis patch grows and starts itching so much that I will scratch it until it bleeds. When I'm extremely stressed, it morphs into a rash that spreads up and down my entire right leg.

"Ewwww...sounds like you need a cream for that!"

I have a cream for it. It's a prescription steroid cream, and it works wonders. As soon as I apply it, my psoriasis clears right up. But a steroid is a potent anti-inflammatory, and the fact that it works so well underscores the fact that something is seriously "off" inside my body. There's an underlying root cause for my inflammation, and over the years, I've determined that my inflammatory trigger is STRESS – usually related to over-work and under-rest.

Personally, I don't want to limit my treatment to slapping on a bandage (i.e. a prescription steroid cream); rather, I want to get to the bottom of the issue. Uncovering – and then taking seriously and treating – the root cause of my condition is the only way for me to truly heal.

Check in with yourself: Can you think of any physical symptom(s) in your life that might be related to stress?

In our "always on, always connected" culture, you need to determine how much is too much for you, remembering that every woman – and every woman's tolerance level – is different. Take an inventory of your life and be realistic. Are you able to juggle all of your roles and tasks without negative implications on your physical, emotional, or spiritual self? If not, you might need to ask for help.

Here's another question to consider in relation to stress: Are you an extravert or an introvert? In other words, does social connection and external stimulation charge you, or does it drain you? If you're an introvert, you might find that continuously being around others – either in person or online – is a stressor. No matter how much you love your friends or co-workers, social interaction can be energetically and emotionally exhausting for introverts. You might feel a strong need to be alone after social events or even after a long day of work or school. It's perfectly okay – and even necessary, for introverts – to respect that need! Furthermore, constant connection via social media, smartphones, and other electronic devices (computers, tablets, etc.) that allow multiple streams of input and information at any one time might be too much for an introvert's energy levels. For some women it works, but for others, it doesn't. Similar to a vegan diet; it works for some people, but definitely not for everybody.

In a similar vein, are you an empath? An "empath" is a character trait commonly observed in women. Empaths have a special ability to intuitively feel and perceive others, and they literally absorb the energy of those around them, sometimes even taking on the emotional and/or physical conditions of others. Empaths feel the emotions (or physical distress) of others and can take these burdens as their own.

If you are an empath, you have to be aware of guarding your own energy and choosing how much energy you want to let in (and from whom, and when). You don't have to become a hermit and stop associating with others, but you do need to place a high priority on your own self-care and allow yourself plenty of space and time after interactions that have a strong energetic exchange.

"I don't think I'm an introvert or an empath, but I still don't understand my crazy-high stress level. Men have always worked and juggled family and other external commitments, so why am I feeling so anxious and stressed about my schedule?"

First, men have never really had to answer the question of, "How do you obtain work-life balance?" It's generally understood and societally accepted that their priorities are more on the "work" side and less on the "family and connections" side. Let's be honest: how often does your male partner take the initiative to send Christmas cards or remember family birthdays? But women, especially women who work outside of the home, often feel exquisite pressure to maintain BALANCE between their external working world and their internal family, home life, and social life. It's a bit skewed.

Another reason women are likely to feel stress more acutely than men is – literally – in our heads. The answer lies within our brains and the fascinating differences between female and male brain anatomy and physiology. *The New Feminine Brain,* by Dr. Mona Lisa Schulz, offers an in-depth explanation of these differences and the impact they have on our innate abilities, strengths, and weaknesses. In a nutshell, the traditional female brain has more neural connections between brain areas and more connectivity in general. This means that we're more likely to think about multiple things at once. It also means we have a greater capacity for growth and change over time (neural plasticity). Great, right? Well, most of the time. Unfortunately, this higher connectivity is another reason why women are more susceptible to distractibility, depression, mood disorders, and anxiety.[31]

Why are traditional male and female brains so different? Because hundreds of thousands of years ago, the male brain adapted to perform highly focused tasks, such as hunting and protection, while the female brain evolved to handle more diversified simultaneous tasks such as childcare, gathering food, maintaining the living space, and nurturing connections within the family and the tribe. If you like visuals, female brains are like a superhighway with multiple lanes and branching on- and off-ramps, whereas male brains are a simple highway overpass.

In *The New Feminine Brain*, Dr. Schulz states, "In the traditional male brain, one issue appears on the neural screen at a time." That's not true for women. Schulz explains, "In the traditional female brain, many issues appear on your mental screen simultaneously. The kids, the pets, the job, the taxes, the upcoming payroll, the lawn, a possible war, the abducted teenager in the news, all of it."[31]

Whereas the traditional male brain opens a single (mental) file at a time, deals with it, and then closes it, the traditional female brain is a bit more like a mad scientist in a crazy chemistry lab. She runs the risk of being a little bit scattered, but she's a genius in her ability to see the big picture. She compares information, understands it as a whole, makes associations and inferences, and has the capacity for a strong sense of intuition.

Interestingly, and in large part due to the superior neural plasticity of the feminine brain, female brains are changing. Modern women are now displaying traits of a more traditionally masculine brain. **However, in most cases, our bodies still haven't caught up to this evolutionary**

cerebral remodeling. Our hormones still go haywire when our brain signals indicate stress. We might very well have the MENTAL capacity to handle the stress, but our bodies aren't "there" yet.

The upshot is this: if you spend your day at work, surrounded by people, projects, and mental stimulation, come home to a family who demands your time and attention, and then "unwind" to social media while simultaneously watching the television, you may be overloading your über-connected feminine brain, especially if you tend toward introversion or characteristics of an empath.

It is essential for your health and happiness to get real with yourself about your capacity for external input, commitments, responsibilities, and physical and emotional stress. **Why? Because stress robs you of creativity, of your libido, and of your energy.** Chronic stress makes you age more rapidly, it packs on the pounds due to the belly-fat storage effects of stress hormones, it can make you want to withdraw from friends and loved ones, it can cause you to lose sleep, and it can even contribute to adrenal fatigue and autoimmunity (more info coming).

Get honest, and then take action. If you're feeling overwhelmed you don't need to eliminate your stressors entirely, but you do need to take inventory. Identify what can be released or shifted in order to reduce stress. Ask for help. Learn how to say "no."

As author and speaker Danielle LaPorte states, "Busy is most often a choice." She goes on to state, "Whatever is on your plate got there because you said yes to it – in the fullness of ambition and desire and wanting to eat life whole."[32] This is not always a bad thing, but it can get rancid fast if "wanting to eat life whole" starts eating you up on the inside. Since everything on your (metaphorical) plate is there because you put it there, you have the power to take it off. It is essential to know your limits and to voice them by saying, "I'm sorry, but no. I can't do that [now, anymore, ever again]."

Now that we've explored our brains and stress, did you know that low-fat diets can also be a culprit when it comes to our ability to handle and manage stress? It's true. Let's talk about dietary fat (and more) in the next section, "Hormone Imbalance and Adrenal Fatigue."

HORMONE IMBALANCE AND ADRENAL FATIGUE

As Dr. Sara Gottfried, author of *The Hormone Cure*, writes, "It's not fair but it's a fact: women are much more vulnerable to hormonal imbalance than men."[33] Hypothyroid disorder affects women up to fifteen times more often than men, and women feel more stressed than men (indicating stress hormone imbalance). Gottfried cites that 26% of women in the US are medicated for anxiety, depression, or a general feeling of being unable to cope compared to only 15% of men.[33]

Women are extremely sensitive to hormonal changes. Why? One reason is that we have babies, and pregnancy increases the demands on our endocrine (hormone producing) glands. Add to this the stress of juggling multiple roles (mother, wife, employee, etc.), and you have a recipe for strain on your organ reserve. Your organ reserve is the ability of your organs – such as your ovaries, thyroid, adrenals, and liver – to withstand life's demands and to restore balance in your body. Unfortunately, your organ reserve naturally declines as you age. According to Gottfried, "After age thirty, organ reserve decreases by 1 percent per year, so that by age eighty-five, organ reserve is a fraction of the original capacity." [33]

When your organs are strong and your hormones are in balance, you look and feel your best. When your hormones are out of whack, which is surprisingly common, they can make your life miserable! The great news is that the way you eat, move, think, relax, and sleep can help bring them back into balance naturally.

The hormone story is HUGE. It is the subject of an entirely different book, and not within the scope of *Lady Bits*. **But it's important to note that many hormone imbalances present as lingering conditions or annoyances typically associated with aging, when in reality, they can be often by fixed or improved by managing stress, improving gut health, and getting more sleep.** If you have lingering fatigue, mood swings, or notice a change in your appearance that your intuition tells you to check out, DO IT. Don't ignore your intuitive genius. Stay up-to-date on your annual medical appointments, and if needed, request tests to check your hormone levels.

Before moving on, I want to briefly address two important concepts that women should know about: cholesterol (and why eating a diet that's too low in fat and animal products can be harmful for some women), and adrenal fatigue.

Many of your sex hormones are derived from cholesterol.
Cholesterol! Isn't that wild? For so long, we've been warned to skip the (egg) yolks and to avoid cholesterol at all costs. However, this dietary advice – when taken to the extreme – may actually be costing us our delicate female hormone balance. Our bodies use cholesterol to produce pregnenolone – also known as the "mother hormone" – which is a hormone precursor from which other hormones are made, primarily progesterone and DHEA. Pregnenolone can also make cortisol. When you're chronically stressed, your body makes extra cortisol (the main stress hormone). In order to make more cortisol, your body "steals" from pregnenolone, causing it to produce **more cortisol** and **less of the other hormones**. This "pregnenolone steal" means that progesterone and other hormone levels may fall.[33] If you're eating an extremely low-fat, low-cholesterol diet that doesn't provide your body with enough of the hormonal building blocks (cholesterol) in the first place, this "steal" is going to impact you doubly.

So go ahead...eat (pasture-raised) egg yolks, organic butter, and grass-fed red meat. As long as these foods come from high quality sources and are consumed in moderation, they can actually be supportive of your health and hormones.

Now let's discuss adrenal fatigue. Adrenal fatigue is something that many women have heard about, but it's not well-understood or accepted, especially among practitioners of traditional Western medicine. One theory of adrenal fatigue – which is also known as "burnout" and is identified by symptoms ranging from debilitating fatigue to feeling "tired but wired" and being unable to sleep at night – is that in response to chronic stress, cortisol is first OVER-produced by the adrenals and then ultimately UNDER-produced once the adrenals are "shot."

Christine, a client in her mid-fifties, is an extremely energetic high school teacher. She teaches several Advanced Placement math classes, is the student council advisor, runs the student store, heads up the prom committee, and organizes (and raises funds for) an annual field trip to Greece for 30 of her advanced math students. Christine does all of this is in addition to mothering two teenagers with a husband who's often away on business. Christine states, "I never – I mean NEVER – felt like things were 'too much' for me until a few years ago. Then all of the sudden it hit. I was completely overwhelmed and stressed out, and I realized that something had to give."

After some thought and prioritization, Christine states, "I could still do most of the things I wanted to do, I just had to do them DIFFERENTLY." She asked for more help at home and at school, she let go of a few of the tasks and commitments that weren't necessary, and she realized the value of listening to her body and honoring her need for a break. Christine says, "I'm getting older. I can't keep the same pace that I kept when I was in my twenties. And that's okay!"

It's possible that Christine finally "hit a wall" and compromised her adrenals. Thankfully, she slowed down before symptoms progressed too far.

Nora Gedgaudas, a nutritional consultant, clinical neurofeedback specialist, and international best-selling author, has another take on adrenal fatigue. She states that adrenal fatigue is a complex issue in which the natural cortisol rhythm is "out of sync." Normally, cortisol is highest in the morning and falls to its lowest levels in the evening. Gedgaudas states that this natural circadian rhythm changes in people with symptoms of adrenal fatigue; they may over-produce cortisol, under-produce cortisol, or display an inverse rhythm in which cortisol is lowest in the morning and highest in the evening. She says, "There is an increasing number of people who are producing cortisol at inappropriate amounts, at inappropriate times of the day" and relates these patterns to a rollercoaster. Gedgaudas states that these "out of sync" rhythms may have less to do with the adrenals' ability to produce cortisol and more to do with the brain's response to stress.[34]

In a recent interview, Gedgaudas recommended that people request the Adrenal Stress Index – a salivary hormone test – if they suspect adrenal-related issues, "and that they look at these rhythms and see how normal these rhythms actually look for them." She states:

"If they're rollercoaster-looking, that's not a good sign; that's a sign that part of the mechanism in your brain that normally mitigates those rhythms is failing, and it's typically failing because that part of the brain has lost its integrity and is experiencing degenerative changes… You have to take that very seriously and address this from a brain-based level as opposed to just running out and taking a bunch of adrenal supplements." [34]

The great news is that eating a "clean" unprocessed diet, managing stress, increasing the amount of sleep you're getting on a daily basis, and often REDUCING the amount of high intensity, high-impact exercise you're doing, can start you on the path toward healing from adrenal fatigue. Talk to your healthcare provider – ultimately an integrative practitioner or functional medicine specialist – for more information specific to your needs.

I recommend Gottfried's book, *The Hormone Cure*, for more information about hormone dysfunction and adrenal fatigue, and Nora Gedgaudas's book, *Rethinking Fatigue*, for additional insight.

Adrenal fatigue is real, it's something that should not be dismissed, and it affects millions of women worldwide. Furthermore, keeping your adrenals strong and healthy when you're pre-menopausal is essential, as your adrenals become the main hormone "factory" in your body after menopause. Do what you can to protect your adrenals NOW so that you can maintain sufficient adrenal reserve throughout your life.

AUTOIMMUNE AND THYROID DISORDERS

We live in a world of vaccines, hand sanitizer, bleach, and safety precautions.

On our plastic playground equipment children are highly unlikely to get a splinter, and with our rubberized playground mats a fall may result in an "ouch," but probably won't create a skinned knee. All of this is good, to a point... But what happens when our immune system is no longer called upon to fight the normal germs and scrapes of growing up? It becomes dysregulated, and sometimes it goes a little crazy.

Ladies, listen up! Autoimmune diseases – a varied group of illnesses in which the body's immune system becomes misdirected and attacks its own organs, from skin to joints to endocrine and gastrointestinal systems – affect three times more women than men. Named a "major women's health issue" by the National Institutes of Health, autoimmunity is the underlying cause of more than 100 serious, chronic illnesses and affects 50 million Americans, more than 75 percent of them being women.[35]

Autoimmune diseases are responsible for more that $100 billion in direct healthcare costs annually. You may have heard of Systemic Lupus Erythematosus (usually referred to as SLE or lupus), but did you know that Rheumatoid Arthritis (RA), and Multiple Sclerosis (MS) are also autoimmune disorders? Each of these diseases affects far more women than men, in ratios of 9:1 (lupus), 2.5:1 (RA), and 2:1 (MS).[35]

I mentioned the thyroid in the previous section on hormones; an estimated **20 million Americans** have some form of thyroid disease, and **one in eight women** will develop a thyroid disorder during her lifetime.[36] Hypothyroidism is one of the most common thyroid disorders, characterized by mental slowing, depression, dementia, weight gain, constipation, dry skin, hair loss, cold intolerance, hoarse voice, irregular menstruation, infertility, muscle stiffness and pain, and a wide range of other symptoms...even surprising symptoms such as thinning in the outer third of the eyebrows!

Studies show that 90% of people with hypothyroidism are producing antibodies to thyroid tissue (this is known as Hashimoto's Thyroiditis).[37] In this situation, the antibodies attack the thyroid tissue causing less thyroid hormone to be produced. The standard plan of care is to supplement with thyroid hormone, but this doesn't address the underlying cause: the fact that the immune system is out of control and attacking the body's own tissues. As licensed acupuncturist, holistic nutritionist, and intrepid researcher Chris Kresser states, "[Prescription] thyroid hormones are like bailing water [in a leaky rowboat]. They may be a necessary part of the treatment. But unless the immune dysregulation is addressed (plugging the leaks), whoever is in that boat will be fighting a losing battle to keep it from sinking."[38] In other words, although prescription thyroid hormone might be a necessary component of the overall treatment plan, medications don't address the root cause. Kresser goes on to state:

*"What the vast majority of hypothyroidism patients need to understand is that they don't have a problem with their thyroid, **they have a problem with their immune system** attacking the thyroid. This is crucial to understand, because when the immune system is out of control, it's not only the thyroid that will be affected."* [38]

One leading explanation for WHY autoimmunity is so prevalent is based on food sensitivities and the resulting inflammation that builds up over time. Essentially, over-exposing your body to a food that it is sensitive to can create antibodies to the food. These antibodies are then misdirected and end up attacking your own body's tissues. Gluten can be a culprit, and for many people (myself included), gluten is something that needs to be avoided. But anything that is seen as "foreign" by your body and yet is continuously introduced (whether this is a food you ingest or an ingredient you apply – for example, a lotion that you rub into your skin every day), can create antibodies and the possibility of an autoimmune attack on your body's own tissues.

If you have (or suspect you have) a thyroid or any other autoimmune disorder you need to seek treatment from a qualified healthcare practitioner, preferably a specialist in integrative or functional medicine who will look beyond prescription medication. But just as in the previous section on hormones and adrenal fatigue, there is good news – simple lifestyle changes, such as identifying food intolerances, eating a "clean" unprocessed diet, minimizing toxic load, managing stress, and increasing the amount of sleep you're getting on a daily basis, can help treat – and may even help resolve – certain autoimmune and thyroid conditions. The *Lady Bits* program is a great place to start!

For more detailed information about a natural approach to treating autoimmune disease, I highly recommend *The Paleo Approach: Reverse Autoimmune Disease and Heal Your Body* by Sarah Ballantyne, who earned a Ph.D. in medical biophysics and spent years researching innate immunity and inflammation before healing her own autoimmune disorders through lifestyle management.

OSTEOPENIA AND OSTEOPOROSIS

We've all known (or had) a grandmother with posture so stooped that her chin nearly touched her chest, or an elderly relative who took a seemingly minor slip in the tub and ended up breaking her hip resulting in hospitalization, surgery, and weeks – or even months – of rehab. For some people, osteoporosis heralds the onset of a loss of independence.

Osteoporosis, a disease in which bone mineral density has decreased to the point that the bones are brittle and at high risk for breaking, is a common condition among both men and women…but especially women. Osteoporosis affects at least 30% of women and 12% of men at some point in their life.[39]

Osteopenia is the precursor to osteoporosis. Bone mineral density (BMD) tests called DEXA scans use X-rays to measure how many grams of calcium and other minerals are packed into a segment of bone. Osteopenia – defined as a BMD T-score between negative 1.0 and negative 2.5 – is an indication that your BMD is below normal.[40] A diagnosis of osteopenia is basically a big, flashing yellow "caution" signal, meaning that your BMD is somewhat lower than "normal," but not low enough to be considered osteoporosis…yet.

The scary thing is that osteopenia and osteoporosis are "silent" and relatively painless. Many women have osteoporosis and never find out, or only find out after breaking a bone.

What can you do to prevent osteopenia (and its more advanced form, osteoporosis)? Plenty. First, let's talk about calcium.

I am leery about relying on calcium supplements due to the possibility that they may increase the risk of cardiovascular disease.[41] Thankfully, the calcium found in foods that are naturally calcium-rich is always safe. The following are some examples of food-based sources of calcium:

- White beans and black-eyed peas (consider soaking and/ or sprouting legumes to make them more digestible and to reduce levels of phytic acid, which can inhibit absorption of calcium)

- Canned salmon and sardines (calcium-rich largely because of the bones, which are small and edible since they soften during the canning process)

- Dried figs

- Blackstrap molasses

- Almonds (like legumes, consider soaking and/or sprouting nuts to make them more digestible and to reduce levels of phytic acid)

- Oranges

- Dark green leafy greens, particularly collards, turnip greens, mustard greens, bok choy, and kale

- Sesame seeds and tahini (sesame seed paste)

- Hemp seeds

- Seaweed

- Broccoli

- Bone broth

Organic dairy from pasture-raised cows, sheep, or goats (recommended only if you are not dairy-sensitive; some people tolerate fermented dairy products such as yogurt or kefir more easily than milk and/or cheese)

You also need to be sure that you are ABSORBING the calcium you ingest. If you are intolerant to a certain food that you consistently eat – for example, gluten – your gut lining will become inflamed over time. An inflamed, angry gut will have difficulty absorbing and assimilating the calcium you bring into your body no matter how much of the "good stuff" you eat.

This was the case for my mother. She was diagnosed with osteopenia via a DEXA scan. Soon after, she tested positive for gluten intolerance, and subsequently removed gluten entirely from her diet. **A year later, when retested with a DEXA scan, her bone mineral density had improved to the point that she was no longer osteopenic.** This had everything to do with inflammation. Before removing gluten from her diet, her guts were irritated, grumpy, and unable to absorb calcium. After removing gluten, her (much happier) guts could relax, recover, and begin to absorb and assimilate the nutrients necessary for strong bones.

Of course, you need more than high-calcium foods alone.

Fat-soluble vitamins A, D, and K2, and the mineral magnesium are essential for proper calcium absorption. Consume egg yolks for vitamin A, consider grass-fed butter or ghee and naturally fermented sauerkraut for vitamin K2, consider magnesium supplementation as needed, and spend time outside as an excuse to make vitamin D.

Speaking of vitamin D, did you know that it is actually a hormone? That being said, you also need to keep your hormonal pathways in balance by getting enough sleep, **managing your stress**, and keeping your blood sugar stable and under control.

It always seems to come back to stress, doesn't it? In *The Slow Down Diet*, Marc David explains that STRESS can actually cause a leeching of calcium out of the bones.42 David is a proponent of **deep breathing** when it comes to stress management and overall wellness, and so am I! Conscious, deep breathing is a wonderful, health-promoting (and possibly even bone-building) practice.

Take a deep breath right now.

Finally, great bone health requires plenty of **weight-bearing exercise using proper posture and alignment** to physically stress (and ultimately, strengthen) your load-bearing joints, which are the joints most often affected by osteoporosis.

Since bone mass peaks in your twenties, the key is to move, move, and then move some more in order to build strong bones that will protect you into old age. If you're beyond your twenties, all is not lost! Keep on moving, walking regularly, doing exercises such as those found in this book, and consider the following:

- Extension exercises are excellent for the health of the vertebrae (for example, cobra pose in yoga, and the "superwoman" exercise found in the Inner Core Energizer routine). The act of spinal extension utilizes muscles that insert into the spine. These muscles essentially "tug" on the vertebrae, thereby gently stressing the bones, which in turn, builds bone density.

- The numerous hip and gluteal (butt) strengthening exercises in the Inner Core Energizer are also excellent for preventing osteoporosis, since many of these muscles attach into the femur (thigh) bone in regions that tend to be weak in people with osteoporosis. The more these muscles tug on the bone, the stronger the bones will become.

- Just like any part of the body, "use it or lose it." The same goes for bone health! You must stress your bones via muscular action and weight-bearing exercises (moving around when you're upright), or else the bones will weaken and become brittle no matter how much calcium you ingest.

- If you enjoy yoga, consider disciplines of yoga that involve holding poses for 60 seconds or longer. Many forms of **hatha yoga** require longer hold times, and the teachers focus on proper alignment (which, again, is essential when it comes to healthy bone-building).

From decreasing your risk of chronic disease to building stronger bones, there are numerous reasons to eat clean, move daily, and manage stress. Let's talk about another – sex.

LOW LIBIDO AND OTHER SEXUAL DIFFICULTIES

If you don't desire sex the way you used to, you are in good company. A recent large-scale study (including almost 32,000 females age 18 and older) found that overall, 43.1% of women reported some kind of sexual problem. A whopping 39% reported diminished sexual desire, 26% reported problems with arousal, and 21% reported problems with achieving orgasm. The most distress occurred among mid-life women.[43]

The article reporting this study included an interview with Sheryl Kingsberg, chief of the division of behavioral medicine at MacDonald Women's Hospital in Cleveland, Ohio. Kingsberg stated:

"This is a wake-up call to health-care professionals . . . of the importance of sexual health and sexual quality of life. Forty percent of patients have sexual concerns, and 12 percent have enough of a concern that it's a significant dysfunction in life. This needs to be addressed." [43]

I completely agree. If this study is representative of the average American woman, then millions of American women are affected, and hundreds of millions of women world wide could also be affected. The great news is that through knowing your body, loving yourself, keeping your inner core muscles strong and fit, and a few simple tricks described in Part VI, feeling sexual desire (and having great sex) is possible again.

PELVIC PAIN AND DYSPAREUNIA (PAINFUL SEX)

If you suffer from dyspareunia, or pain with intercourse, please seek help from a qualified women's health physical therapist or other specialized healthcare provider. Dyspareunia is a fairly common condition and, unfortunately, it is frequently left untreated since many women are embarrassed to talk about it, ashamed of their condition, or left to think that it's "normal" for sex to be painful. Women who suffer from dyspareunia may not want to have sex, but often feel obligated to participate for the sake of their partner.

If you have dyspareunia you may have brought the issue up with your healthcare provider and been left to think that it's all "in your head" (it is not) or that the condition will resolve on its own (it may or may not). You may feel like your provider does not care or is not listening to you, but in actuality he or she may not be aware of the symptoms of dyspareunia or the broader category of pelvic pain that often contributes to painful intercourse – chronic pelvic pain syndrome, or CPPS. CPPS is a mystery to many healthcare providers because the cause is not often clear and the symptoms can vary widely.

CPPS can result from a variety of factors, including traumatic injury, such as car accidents or falls, injuries sustained during pregnancy or childbirth, a history of painful periods or endometriosis, a history of chronic urinary tract infections or yeast infections, interstitial cystitis (painful bladder syndrome), psychological trauma, or a history of physical or sexual abuse. Often it is a combination of multiple issues: the culmination of a complicated gynecological and/or psychosocial history that results in overactive, painful pelvic floor muscles. Overactive pelvic floor muscles make intercourse painful. Painful intercourse leads to anxiety about intercourse, which leads to more muscle tension and more pain.

Does this strike a chord with you? Initially, you may not think twice about your own gynecological or pelvic history but when you put all the pieces together you may realize, **"I really have been through a lot!"**

I have worked with many women with CPPS who have histories that sound something like this:

"When I was fifteen I fell off a horse and landed on my tailbone. I couldn't walk for over a week. Then when I was seventeen I had a huge ovarian cyst that ruptured and sent me to the emergency room. Afterward, I kept having pain in my lower abdomen, and my gynecologist recommended exploratory laparoscopic surgery. Turns out I had endometriosis, and over the next five years I had three additional surgeries to remove endometrial lesions.

Luckily I was still able to have kids! My first son weighed eight pounds and I tore badly… My second pregnancy was a miscarriage. My third pregnancy resulted in an emergency C-section because I was nearly two weeks late and the baby was huge – and breech. I had a hysterectomy last year because of a uterine fibroid and my surgeon said I had a ton of scar tissue in the abdomen and pelvis... Do you think any of this contributes to the pain I experience during sex?"

Do I think her history contributes to her pain? Yes! This fictional patient – although similar to multiple women I have worked with – has dealt with pathological trauma from endometriosis and a ruptured ovarian cyst, physical trauma from the fall, three pregnancies and two (difficult) live births, scarring from multiple surgeries, and emotional trauma from the miscarriage. It is likely that a pelvic examination would reveal tension and tenderness in the pelvic floor, possibly muscle spasm, and probably weakness. Her pelvic floor muscle dysfunction causes sex to be painful, which creates anxiety and reactive muscle tension related to sex. This causes global muscular tension during intimacy, particularly in the pelvic floor region, which in turn creates even more pain during intercourse... And the cycle continues.

If this could be your story, please seek help. Do not feel like you need to be "strong" about the pain – it may not resolve on its own. **Study and take to heart the information about relaxation that is provided in Chapter 11. Focus on the stretching exercises rather than the strengthening exercises, and do not complete kegels in any form if they cause pain or discomfort.**

It is important to find a healthcare practitioner who is sympathetic to your condition. A multidisciplinary approach can be incredibly helpful. This should include – at the very least – a gynecologist (or certified nurse midwife, nurse practitioner, or naturopath) and a women's health physical therapist (WHPT). You might also consider seeking the services of a psychologist or counselor, and/or treatment from a chiropractor, massage therapist, acupuncturist, or holistic nutritionist. Sometimes medication will be prescribed such as antidepressants, muscle relaxants, or topical creams to dull the pain.

My advice with a multidisciplinary approach is to start with the essentials for conservative treatment (i.e. a gynecologist and a WHPT), then add additional disciplines one at a time so that you know what

Lady Bits

works and what does not. Jumping into ten different types of therapy at the same time is overwhelming and may not be effective. For example, if you are working with a physical therapist, massage therapist, acupuncturist, herbalist, and psychologist and notice a change in your condition, you will not know which treatment(s) contributed to the change unless you systematically add them in, one by one.

On a separate but related note, I am a firm believer that – unless you have an emergent situation or a specific pathology that requires it – surgery should be avoided until conservative treatment options have been exhausted. **In short, if you have dyspareunia, there is help for you.** For many individuals, the treatment can be as simple as basic stretching and relaxation training...not as complex or risky as "going under the knife."

"Just to clarify – physical therapy can help with painful sex? How?"

Absolutely! Physical therapists are highly trained professionals (often with a doctorate in physical therapy – DPT) who are experts at evaluating the musculoskeletal system. Physical therapists who specialize in women's health have been specially trained to diagnose and treat conditions associated with pelvic floor dysfunction. **If you have been referred to a WHPT and you are wondering what to expect, read on.**

Your WHPT will ask you detailed questions about your current complaints and your history, including your medical and gynecological history, social history, past history of injuries, and your lifestyle. She will want to know specifics about any difficulties you are having, from functional activities that have become difficult to social issues you are experiencing due to your problem. Do not leave anything out! Some of the most important details that helped me (as a WHPT) diagnose and develop an appropriate plan of care came from remarks patients made as an afterthought, stating, "I don't know if this matters, but..." **Usually, it does matter!**

After the interview is complete and your WHPT has a good understanding of your history and current condition, she will move on to a physical examination. Your WHPT will screen your back and hips for any impairments that might contribute to your pain, evaluate your posture, and complete a pelvic examination. The pelvic examination is a very important component of the initial (evaluative) visit. It is usually completed vaginally and/or rectally after you have consented to the procedure. Although it may feel uncomfortable and embarrassing, keep in mind that your WHPT has had extensive training in the pelvic examination procedure specifically for the evaluation and treatment of the pelvic floor muscles and the surrounding tissues. The pelvic examination helps your WHPT assess your current level of pelvic floor muscle pain and tension and allows her to begin treatment with manual therapy techniques such as trigger point release and/or stretching.

In addition to manual therapy techniques completed in-clinic, dilator therapy may be prescribed. This involves progressive stretching of the pelvic floor muscles using a tool called a dilator. Dilator therapy is a great adjunct to in-clinic treatment because it can be done at home, in a relaxed setting, with or without your partner.

Relaxation training is an essential component of physical therapy treatment since dyspareunia is a cycle that starts and ends with pain. Pain makes the muscles tense, which causes more pain, which causes more muscular tension, which causes more pain…and on and on. Your WHPT will help interrupt this cycle so that you can recover and move forward from the pain cycle that can be so debilitating.

Always keep the lines of communication flowing. Ask your WHPT any questions that arise, and voice any concerns or discomfort you may have. Open communication is imperative when it comes to successful treatment of pelvic floor dysfunction.

Remember, you are not alone if you suffer from pain that makes sex difficult or impossible. It is not your fault, it is not a flaw, and **there is help**.

PREMENSTRUAL SYNDROME (PMS)

I have to admit – when I was younger, I didn't believe in PMS. I didn't experience painful periods or mood issues until my son was born. After his birth, I experienced mild PMS: mood swings, cramps, and food cravings...the typical "stuff." Annoying, but not severe enough to classify as horrendous. But then, in my mid-thirties (as I described in the introduction of this book), PMS hit me like a freight train. I will never, ever, EVER dismiss PMS as "imaginary" again.

From PMS to perimenopause and on into menopause, hormonal ups and downs can wreak havoc on a woman's life.

But did you know that it's possible for a period to sneak up on you without you even being aware? To have it start WITHOUT cramps that cause you to double over in fetal position, sometimes bad enough to induce nausea, chills, back pain, or pain that radiates down your legs? For me, significant – almost miraculous – relief has come in the form of stress management, yoga, and relaxation, but there are other keys that might help you as well. Let's discuss a few of the latest findings.

If you have been following the conversation so far, you probably have an inkling that it's (almost) this simple: decrease gut inflammation and manage your stress, and everything will improve. It's true! Heal your guts, heal your brain, heal your hormones... Heal your life.

The brain depends on gut bacteria for protection, since the gut microbiota produce neurotransmitters including serotonin and dopamine. Serotonin and dopamine are important mood regulators, and having adequate levels of them is more important than ever when our hormones fluctuate (as they naturally do, every menstrual cycle).

We've discussed the problem with eating foods that your body doesn't tolerate: it can damage your gut, potentially leading to autoimmune disease and widespread inflammation. Unchecked food sensitivities can cause all manner of mental and physical health issues. Thus, one very important thing you can do to limit or even eliminate PMS is to identify foods your body is sensitive to, and then stop eating them. Research "elimination diets" and talk to a functional medicine specialist or holistic nutritionist for guidance.

Women's health advocate Dr. Christiane Northrup has additional advice for women. She states that you should limit – but not eliminate – salt intake during the days (or weeks) when you typically experience PMS. Limiting salt will reduce bloating all over the body, including water retention in the brain. This may ease both physical and emotional symptoms.[44]

Northrup also encourages cutting out sugar and limiting caffeine, both of which can make PMS symptoms worse. **But don't eliminate sugar and coffee and then substitute caffeinated diet soft drinks instead!** Diet sodas often contain aspartame, which is a known excitotoxin (along with monosodium glutamate, or MSG). An excitotoxin is a chemical that makes brain cells shift into overdrive, and may make PMS symptoms worse. [44]

"Now I know what to avoid... Is there anything to add?"

Talk with your doctor about supplementing with B vitamins, and consider food-based approaches to increasing levels of zinc (found in poultry, beef and lamb, seafood such as oysters, nuts and seeds, and mushrooms), and magnesium (found in unsweetened cocoa powder, legumes, nuts and seeds, seafood such as halibut, whole grains such as brown rice and quinoa, and vegetables).

Finally, experts advise women to pay close attention to both weight and exercise, and not to take either one to extremes. "Maintaining a healthy weight – not overweight, not underweight – and exercising regularly, without overdoing it, helps to ease PMS symptoms and make them easier to cope with," says Rebecca Amaru, MD, clinical instructor of obstetrics and gynecology at the Mt. Sinai Medical Center in New York City.[44]

> **Fun Tidbit:** Vaginal steaming (or "yoni steaming") is hot right now...both literally and figuratively! While douching and other forms of cleansing are not necessary (or even recommended) for vaginal health, vaginal steam treatments can be relaxing and rejuvenating for your lady bits. Proponents claim that vaginal steaming can reduce cramping and other symptoms of PMS, relieve symptoms of menopause, aid in fertility, and assist with

the healing of hemorrhoids (among other benefits).

To give this time-honored treatment a try, you will need water, herbs such as rosemary, basil, lavender, rose petals, chamomile, and/or dandelion, a basin, two blankets, and a seating setup (options described below). Simply add a handful of herbs to your basin, and then pour very hot water into the basin until it is nearly full. Test the temperature of the steam with your forearm. Your genitals are very sensitive, and you don't want to burn them, so do NOT sit over the steam bath until the temperature is comfortable!

Remove your underwear and sit over the basin using your preferred seating setup. Some seating options:

- Place the basin into the bowl of your toilet (you'll need an exact fit to do this) and sit on your toilet seat as you usually would.

- Squat over the basin if it is shallow enough and if you're comfortable holding a deep squat for a long period of time.

- Use a special vaginal steaming stool (crafted with a hole in the middle of the seat to allow the steam to rise through).

- Probably the most realistic option: Find a chair with a slatted seat made of natural materials (for example, a slatted wooden deck chair) and place the basin below it.

If you don't have a slatted chair, set up two chairs side-by-side about six inches apart. Place a cutting board on the rungs between the two chairs, and place the basin on the cutting board. Sit with a cheek on each chair, with the basin directly below.

Regardless of your seating setup, be sure the steam isn't too close to your genitals; you don't want to burn yourself. Wrap yourself in blankets (one up high and one tenting around your steaming setup) – and relax for 20-30 minutes. This is a great time for meditation, listening to calming music, journaling, or reading uplifting material. When you're done with the steam, rise slowly, remain wrapped in your blankets, and then settle into bed for a nap or for the night.

NOTE: Do not try this at home if you are pregnant or think you might be, as certain herbs have been known to induce labor and may be contra-indicated for certain health or medical conditions. You may also need to avoid vaginal steaming if you have an IUD. If you have any doubts about whether or not vaginal steaming is suitable for you, or which herbs to use, consult your physician, naturopathic doctor, or integrative medical practitioner.[45, 46]

PERIMENOPAUSE

It can start as early as your thirties or as late as your fifties: the life change known as perimenopause, a time when your hormones shift, egg production dwindles, and you can feel like you're losing your mind. Some women feel like they're becoming a different woman altogether, which can be disconcerting or celebratory – but always interesting. Perimenopause can last for quite a long time (ten years or more),

"I'm not there yet. What should I expect?"

Due to fluctuating hormone levels, you might notice warm flashes, hot flashes, or SUPER-HOT hot flashes! You might feel moody, foggy, forgetful, and lethargic. A perimenopausal client told me, "Some mornings when I open my eyes, my eyelids seem to stay shut." The following stories are from clients who have been through perimenopause and come out on the other side.

Meg, now in her mid-fifties:
"Perimenopause for me (age 48-54) was an emotional roller coaster. I over-reacted to things and I never knew who was speaking – my hormones or me. I finally got through the changes last year, and feel like I've calmed down again. The irregular periods were very difficult to manage – some light, some very heavy, and I never knew when they would hit. The hot flashes were so bad that I had to give up coffee and red wine, which didn't help my mood! But my doctor really discouraged estrogen replacement and I toughed it out."

Zhanet, age 57:

"Perimenopause started around age 46 or 47 and it SUCKED! It lasted about ten years and there were mood changes – irritability, increased feelings of stress and anxiety, increased pelvic pain during periods, and periods that wouldn't EVER QUIT – lasting sometimes more than two weeks and then getting another one two weeks or less after that. I also noticed increased acne – weeks at a time when I felt like a teenager again. And let's not leave out the night sweats that would literally soak my pajamas and sheets, poor sleep, intense breast sensitivity/pain that lasted for weeks, and finally, periods that truly seemed like my internals were going through something quite violent. I was medically checked out in that entire region but the final consensus was that I just got a really nasty perimenopause experience (lucky me). I am almost ready to declare having arrived at true menopause. I've been period-free for about nine months, but it needs to be twelve to officially say that I'm menopausal. Now that I have finally reached this period-free stage, it's like the storm has passed and I feel pretty darn great every day: Peaceful, healthy, and relaxed."

What should you do if you hit perimenopause and feel like you've unwittingly entered the highway to Hell? Your first line of defense should be stress management. Like almost every other condition listed in this book, stress can contribute to the discomfort of perimenopause, and can most certainly exacerbate it. We will be discussing stress management in-depth in Chapter 11.

You can also consider making some dietary changes. A 2013 study of over 6,000 women found that consumption of a Mediterranean-style diet decreased the risk of hot flashes and night sweats.[47] Typically, a Mediterranean diet is high in vegetables and healthy fats such as olive oil, moderately high in lean protein (often with an emphasis on fish), and fairly low in sugar. This advice is corroborated by Dr. Christiane Northrup, who advises limiting salt and eliminating refined sugar and white flour; basically, "the white stuff." Northrup also recommends cutting back on caffeine and wine, since some women find that these substances exacerbate perimenopause symptoms.[44]

As far as dietary additions, consider increasing your intake of omega-3 fatty acids (found in salmon, sardines, walnuts, grass-fed beef, and eggs from free-roaming chickens) as well as calcium (see previous section on bone health and note that it is ideal to increase calcium from food-based sources rather than relying on supplements).

MENOPAUSE

Menopause is defined as 12 months or more without a menstrual cycle. Most of my clients who have moved beyond perimenopause into menopause are – overall – quite happy with the outcome. Meg celebrates "no more PMS or cramps or constipation or any of the stuff that goes with a menstrual cycle, which has simplified life! Without little kids around, my back doesn't hurt anymore, and heck...I don't have to pluck my eyebrows because body hair doesn't seem to grow as avidly as it once did!"

On the other hand, other issues can creep in such as fatigue, weight gain, and skin changes. Let's hear from my clients.

Meg:
"I get tired more easily and I like to have some downtime each day. Since menopause, there is a little pad of belly fat that keeps hanging on for dear life. Although I never had to watch my weight, I seem to be gaining five pounds a year over the past few years... ***That's a scary trend****. I've also been surprised at how thin my skin has become. I cut the back of my hand and it took two weeks to heal! And wrinkles – they seem to show up overnight. Ditto age spots. My skin is just looser in general... I didn't know small breasts could sag!"*

Zhanet:
"The dryness of everything – lady parts, skin, eyes, mouth – is sort of irksome and it's apparently not going to go away. It's my new reality. So, I just deal with it. I expected dryness, but I didn't expect it to be all-over-the-body dryness. I didn't expect to see the collapse of my skin and muscles happen so quickly. I didn't expect the word-finding difficulties to start so early and to be so prevalent – but all my same-age pals are going through the same thing, so we can laugh about it together and try to figure out the missing words for each other."

A primary feature of menopause includes changes in the vagina, pelvic floor muscles, and sex drive. Declining estrogen levels can cause thinning of the vaginal and urethral tissues, which can contribute to pain with intercourse. Vaginal tissue thinning, when combined with age-related decline in immune function, leads to an increased potential for skin breakdown and urinary tract infections.

> **Fun Tidbit:** Check your lube! Over-the-counter lubricants can contain endocrine disruptors (parabens such as methylparaben and ethylparaben, as well as phthalates). Endocrine disruptors have been linked to vaginal adenocarcinoma, disorders of ovulation, breast cancer, and uterine fibroids in adult females, as well as disruption of thyroid function, obesity, and diabetes.[48] Safe lubricant options include aloe vera (from the plant itself or in a single-ingredient gel form) or extra virgin oils such as coconut, olive, or jojoba. There is a slight risk of oils getting trapped in the vulvar folds and becoming rancid, so consider cleaning your vulva after lubricating with oils, or perhaps alternate use of oils with aloe vera. If oils and aloe are a little too "natural" for you, Yes® brand vaginal lubricants are pure, paraben-free, and get rave reviews (www.yesyesyes.org).

Many women in perimenopause and menopause struggle with vaginal dryness, and some will notice changes in libido – usually a decrease. However, that's not always the case! Elizabeth states, "I find sex is more enjoyable, but I am not certain if age or wisdom is the contributory factor. Basically, I know what I like." Meg states, "Overall, sex got better once I didn't have to think about pregnancy anymore. And knowing yourself and not being afraid to speak up is a benefit in sex as well as relationships."

Another thing you might experience is that the incidence of urinary incontinence (most notably urge incontinence) increases as women get older. This shift usually begins around the onset of menopause. Aging and menopause do not implicitly cause incontinence; however, age-related changes do increase the risk of developing incontinence **in the absence of specific strengthening exercises and bladder training**

techniques. Some of the age-related changes that typically occur include the following:

- A decrease in elasticity of the smooth muscle fibers of the bladder, which can decrease the bladder's storage capacity.

- The lining of the urethra changes leading to a decrease in compression (and a potential increase in urinary leakage).

- The urethra often becomes less sensitive to sensory input, which may contribute to overactive bladder. [49]

Weakness of the pelvic floor from inadequate exercise can become an issue over time **for women of any age** since disuse of any muscle will lead to muscular atrophy (loss of muscle tissue). Just like the "waddle" that can develop in the triceps (upper arm) region, the pelvic floor muscles become thinner, looser, and less toned if they are not worked regularly.

Moving more doesn't just help the pelvic floor...it's essential for comfort and health of EVERYTHING in your body. Elizabeth states, "I never expected my muscles to tighten up as much as they have or my joints to feel as creaky as they do at times."

Zhanet agrees, but has a solution. She explains:

*"Stiffness is a problem, but it's ten times worse if I take a day off from exercise. I've discovered that **keeping moving** is absolutely essential to me for both physical and mental happiness. I love to exercise alone. During my walks it's my time for self-reflection and meditative moments. While I enjoy exercise classes, I don't have a real need for the group experience in order to keep me going. I'm quite self-disciplined when it comes to exercise, plus I can more easily 'let go' and express myself freely when dancing [Zhanet's workout of choice] if I am alone."*

When asked about the "secret" to lasting health, Zhanet states:

"Health is an ongoing and ever-changing thing. It needs to be reassessed constantly. Your diet, your emotional health, your physical health will change daily in small ways and also over time in bigger ways. You can't ever let

yourself grow complacent about your self-care. It's your body and if you don't look after it, no one else is going to do it for you. Eat well. Eat close to the earth and far from the factories. Try to rely as little as possible on external fixes such as alcohol and medications if you can. Forgive yourself for past mistakes – we all make them. Try to live without hanging on to regrets – you will have regrets, but don't let them eat at you. Let them go and move forward. If you have a sound mind you have a better chance of having a sound body too."

CANCER, HEART DISEASE, AND OTHER FORMS OF CHRONIC ILLNESS

There are numerous chronic diseases that are common – and often devastating – among women. **Know your body, trust your intuition, and make every attempt to take excellent care of your health.** Remember to do your monthly breast self-exams. Keep your annual appointments with your gynecologist and other medical providers. Speak up at the doctor's office. Ask questions. Demand a second opinion if your instincts say so. As my friend Tara (age 34) states:

*"My hysterectomy, to correct a uterine prolapse, was a blessing in disguise. The routine pathology report for my cervix and uterus came back with Stage I uterine cancer – such a shock, although I'd known for over a year that something wasn't right. My doctors believe the hysterectomy got all of the cancer cells, but I will need a Pap in six months and every six months for the next two years, and then every year for the next twenty years. **I am so glad that I know my body because I know when something is 'off.'** I've always been proactive when it comes to reproductive health, and I've made sure to educate myself in that area the best I can. If I didn't know my body so well, things could have been much worse."*

No woman is left behind when it comes to physical changes that occur throughout a lifetime. These inevitable changes require special attention to stress management, proper nutrition, and inner core health and wellness. The fact that you are reading this book is a great start! Keep reading – you're on the right track.

PART IV:
The Proper Care and Feeding of a Female Body

IT'S NOT JUST ABOUT LOOKING GOOD, IT'S ABOUT FEELING GOOD.

*"So many people spend their health gaining wealth,
and then have to spend their wealth to regain their health."*
–A.J. Reb Materi

"The greatest gift you can give your family and the world is a healthy you."
–Joyce Meyer

*"A healthy attitude is contagious but don't wait to catch it from others.
Be a carrier."*
–Tom Stoppard

Good health is simple, although "simple" doesn't necessarily equate to "easy." It takes time, energy, and a mindset shift to properly feed and care for your body, but I'm here to tell you that IT'S WORTH IT. You can look and feel so much better! You can radiate energy and sex appeal and glowing health – and it doesn't have to be a drag. In fact, you can even have some fun with it. Don't just take my word for it...

Alice, 78 years old:
"I consider eating clean and moving every day to be my other health insurance. I wouldn't be as strong as I am now, physically, emotionally, and mentally if I hadn't kept up with exercise and healthy living throughout the years."

Sara, 40 years old:
"I didn't start focusing on my fitness until I was 37. I was never overweight and equated size with health, figuring I was fine and didn't need to worry about exercise. How wrong I was! I started working out on my 37th birthday and got into the best shape of my life, which was good because by the end of the year I was pregnant with baby #4. It was amazing how much easier that pregnancy was, and how much easier my recovery went. I believe it was all due to exercise and nutrition."

We have already discussed the importance of exercise and good nutrition – now it's time for specific action steps. Properly caring for your unique female body is essential for setting a baseline – or foundation – of good health. This foundation will set you up for the remainder of the *Lady Bits* program, which will ultimately lead to a passionate love affair with yourself...with your partner...with your life.

Let's start with sleep.

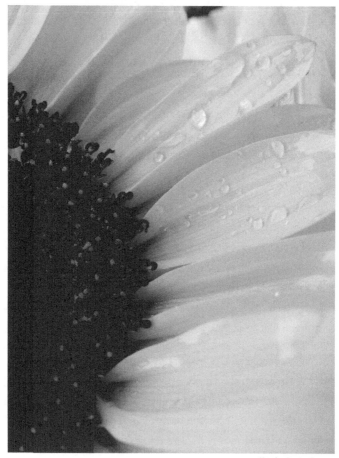

Lady Bits

Chapter 10

SLEEP

Sleep is like your body's housekeeper. All of your bodily systems clean up and detoxify overnight, including the brain, which clears out harmful waste proteins that build up between its cells – a process that may reduce the risk of Alzheimer's disease. As stated in Arianna Huffington's book *Thrive*, you can't "entertain guests" (be awake) and "clean the house" (detoxify during sleep) at the same time.[50]

Remember the adrenal glands? The adrenals need adequate sleep to repair and replenish, and this sleep needs to happen at predictable times. The ideal time for adrenal recovery is 11pm – 1am. For your best shot at capitalizing on the replenishing, detoxifying, stress-relieving benefits of sleep, aim to be in bed by 10pm (or even earlier).

Sleep detoxifies, but sleep **deprivation** changes our brains, our physiology, and our outlook on life. It diminishes our energy and our capacity to make smart choices. This is one reason why sleep loss can lead to weight gain. When you're pooped, why would you want to whip up a healthy snack? Instead, you'll seek quick, easy energy, usually in the form of sugar or a bagel or chips, and then over-indulge without thinking because you CAN'T THINK STRAIGHT. Any sleep-deprived mom can attest to this!

> **"Of all sleep-deprived Americans, women are the most fatigued. Working moms get the least sleep, with 59% of respondents to a national survey reporting sleep deprivation, and 50% saying they get six hours of sleep or less."**
> **–Arianna Huffington, *Thrive*[50]**

You know the feeling that you need to get ONE MORE THING done before bed? Then one thing turns into three or four and pretty soon it's midnight? It's not just you. Many of us are feeling this tug to do MORE, and it seems to be getting worse and worse. One more email comes in that we simply "must" respond to, and once again, sleep gets pushed to the back burner. Sadly, this workaholic mentality leads to lack of sleep, making us less productive, sicker, fatter, and more stressed!

This is not something to be taken lightly. Sleep deprivation is impacting us deeply.

Everything you do, you'll do better with a good night's sleep:

- You'll be less prone to illness, stress, traffic accidents, and weight gain.

- Regular sleep helps you exercise better, longer, safer, and more effectively.

- You'll have more energy and can be more active.

- You'll make better decisions when it comes to your food choices, not to mention choices related to business, family, and house and home.

- You'll look brighter, healthier, and more youthful.

Electric light has shifted our internal clocks such that we're going to bed later than we normally would, and then forcing ourselves to wake up before we're fully rested. This causes a state of chronic sleep deprivation that accumulates over time and becomes sleep debt. As Huffington states, "It's common for people to overeat, but people don't generally oversleep."[50]

What's the solution? **The solution is to stop this madness and make a change.** Here are some of my favorite tips and tricks to help you get sufficient, quality sleep:

- The first is simple, and something you (probably) already do: make your bed daily. I always sleep more soundly in sheets that are smooth and unruffled, and it feels delicious to slip into a neat, tidy bed.

- I also enjoy my silk pillowcase. Silk pillowcases have been said to help decrease facial wrinkles, since they're so slick and smooth.

- The "laptop curfew," which I learned from my mentor Jessica Drummond, is genius. Electronic devices such as computers and even phones and tablets emit blue-spectrum light, which is the daytime spectrum of light. Absorbing this type of light too late in the evening will shift your body's sleep hormones and can disrupt sleep. Set a "laptop curfew" for approximately two hours before bed to help your body adjust and physically prepare for the transition to sleep. Wear blue-blocker glasses if screen time is required at night.

- Schedule sleep like you would a business appointment. Don't blow it off! If you have difficulty making it to your bedroom on time, set an alarm to go off in your bedroom at the appointed hour for sleep. Sometimes getting to your bedroom is half the battle.

- The darker and cooler the room, the better you'll sleep. Cover any LED lights, get room-darkening shades, and use a fan to move the air, keep your room cool, and provide white noise.

- Speaking of temperature, consider sleeping naked. Ditch restrictive nightwear to prevent overheating and allow your body parts to breathe.

- Limit your fluid intake before bed to minimize nighttime "nature calls." Avoid caffeine after 2pm (earlier for some people), and monitor how your body does with alcohol. I've found that as I get older, alcohol either keeps me awake or sometimes wakes me up in the middle of the night – not because I have to go to the bathroom; I simply pop awake and can't get back to sleep. Unfortunately, alcohol is known to disrupt the sleep cycle. It allows for quick entry into deep sleep, but it makes the light sleep (REM sleep) more easily interrupted. So in other words, you'll CRASH...but then you'll wake up during your next REM phase. Many women develop sleep issues as they age, so alcohol's effect may worsen the problem.

If you tend to have difficulty falling asleep, you might want to experiment with supplemental magnesium such as "Natural Calm" made by Natural Vitality. I am not affiliated with this company in any way; I have simply experienced great results in my own life using their products. Magnesium is an essential nutrient that many of us are deficient in, and it may help you sleep more soundly. Talk to your healthcare provider for personalized recommendations based on your nutritional needs.

"What about when I'm lying in bed, wide awake, and I just can't drift off?"

Breathe deeply. No really. Don't just take three or four deep breaths and decide it doesn't work – you've got to give it time. Take at least 10 long, slow, calm breaths. Did you know that when you exhale your heart rate slows down? This is a phenomenon called "respiratory sinus arrhythmia (RSA)." Capitalize on it! Try making your exhales longer than your inhales. If it helps keep your mind on-track, count to 4 as you inhale, hold your breath for 2 counts, and then exhale for 8 counts.

Accept it! I've come to accept and even embrace the fact that sometimes my wild and crazy feminine brain just won't shut down. It does no good to fight it; in fact, stressing over it just makes it more maddening, more stressful, and more difficult to drift away. Settle in, snuggle into your sheets, and say to yourself, "Fun! Let's have a little chat. But let's take it slow and quiet. Let's whisper." For me, this works wonders.

If that doesn't help, get up and grab a bite...something healthy with a balanced ratio of protein, fat, and carbohydrate (for example: half an apple with a drizzle of almond butter). A light midnight snack often does the trick.

Chapter 11

RELAXING, RECHARGING, AND LIVING IN THE MOMENT

"Worry is a prayer for chaos." Take a moment to consider this statement – it's so true! Your thoughts affect your nervous system. Focusing on things that feel negative can take you down in a flash; this is especially for true highly sensitive individuals (in other words, most women).

When it comes to reclaiming your spark in the bedroom and beyond, it is absolutely essential to monitor and protect your energy, breathe deeply, and manage your stress. Easier said than done, right? Well, now is the time to start making stress management a priority. Take care of yourself! You matter.

THE RELAXATION RESPONSE

You can counter the way your body responds to stress by learning how to harness the relaxation response, which indicates an improvement in physiological and psychological markers of stress. When you participate in activities that activate the relaxation response (i.e. meditation, guided visualization, deep breathing, walking or moving with mindfulness, and/or practicing gentle yoga), your heart rate, blood pressure, and breathing rate decrease. Long-term utilization of these practices may result in significant health-related benefits, including the reduced risk of cardiometabolic diseases.[51] Furthermore, as you relax, your body consumes less oxygen and you begin to experience an alteration in your cortical and subcortical brain regions. As feelings of peace and well-being take over, specific changes in gene expression can occur.[52]

You can literally change your brain and your body with the relaxation response. Isn't that amazing?

> "Tension is who you think you should be.
> Relaxation is who you are."
> –Chinese Proverb

Let's begin by focusing on relaxation of the inner core. Ahhhh.... Relaxation. What a yummy word. Allow it to feel delightful and wonderful and not stressful or something you have to grasp or strive for. *Lady Bits* is all about tender love and care of your body and acceptance of where you are NOW, while consistently working toward where you want to be. The first step in learning how to relax is learning how to breathe.

CORE BREATHING

Many people are familiar with diaphragmatic breathing (also known as "belly breathing"), but few people practice it regularly, throughout the day. An excellent goal to work toward is the practice of taking 30 second "breath breaks" every one to two hours. This is an excellent way to promote relaxation throughout the entire body, including the inner core.

"Oh come on... I know how to breathe! I'm alive, aren't I?"

You may know how to breathe in order to sustain life, but most of us do not know how to breathe deeply – yet quietly and calmly – in a way that facilitates total body relaxation. Most of us go through life taking shallow breaths high up in our chests. This over-utilizes the accessory muscles of respiration and underutilizes the one muscle whose sole purpose is quiet, restful breathing: the diaphragm.

The accessory muscles of respiration are primarily neck and shoulder muscles that help to move the collarbones, sternum, and ribcage in order to make more room for lung expansion. They are the muscles that evolved to assist the diaphragm in times of trouble, for example, to outrun a predator. These muscles make our chests heave so that our lungs can really expand for situations that require extra oxygen. They are invaluable when you need them to kick in; however, we don't usually need our chests to heave! Many people use these muscles regardless of activity level resulting in small, shallow breaths from the upper chest.

Unfortunately, overusing these muscles (when unnecessary) can cause them to become overactive and tense.

For most situations in modern life, quiet, diaphragmatic breathing is ideal to meet our respiration requirements. I am going to explain diaphragmatic breathing **with a twist**. In addition to teaching you the basic breathing technique, I will show you how diaphragmatic breathing can allow you to feel and appreciate the muscles of the pelvic floor. As you begin to sense the connection between the pelvic floor (the "floor" of the inner core) and the diaphragm (the "ceiling" of the inner core), your inner core awareness will improve and the mind-body connection will increase. From this point forward, I will refer to this type of diaphragmatic breathing as **Core Breathing**.

EXERCISE – Core Breathing:

Sit comfortably or lie down, and relax your shoulders.

Place hands below your bellybutton, fingertips lightly touching.

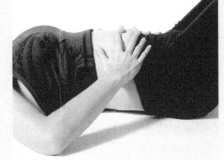

Inhale deeply through your nose and into your abdomen so that your belly and lower ribcage gently expand outward, to the sides, and to the back. You should feel your fingers draw apart (see picture). As the pressure inside your abdomen increases, you will also sense a feeling of gentle downward pressure on your pelvic floor. Allow this downward movement to happen – <u>do not resist it</u>.

Slowly exhale through your mouth as if you are blowing through a straw, and allow your belly to return to the starting position. Sense your pelvic floor gently lifting as the pressure inside your abdomen decreases. This should not feel like a kegel, just a gentle (and very small) upward movement of your pelvic floor.

A great visualization is to imagine a balloon inside your belly. As you inhale, it inflates three-dimensionally, pressing forward into your abdomen, back and sideways into your lower ribs, and down into your pelvic floor. As you exhale, it deflates entirely.

Throughout this practice your upper chest and shoulders should be fairly still. The abdomen is what you will see moving, and in time, you will begin to sense the pelvic floor's gentle movement as well.

Continue to breathe deeply, releasing tension with each exhale. Feel your body "melting."

If you slip out of this breath pattern, do not give up! Just slip back in.

Practice this for as long as you need to in order to get accustomed to it. Practice in different positions (lying down, sitting, standing), and in different situations (alone, with your partner, in a crowded room). Be gentle with yourself. You do not have to take big gulps of air – just breathe normally.

Initially, this can feel strange if you are accustomed to breathing high in the chest. You may feel like you can't get enough oxygen, or like you are struggling for breath. However, with practice and focus this will become second nature and – I assure you – will feel incredibly relaxing.

EXERCISE – Breath Breaks:

Set an alarm on your computer or a timer on your watch to go off every one to two hours. Alternatively, cell phone applications exist for "mindfulness" training that will notify you by sound or vibration to take a moment to breathe, relax, and be in the moment.

Use the alarm as your cue to pause what you are doing and initiate Core Breathing for 30 seconds (or more, if you wish). Allow your mind to clear and your body to melt for 30 seconds. You will only take approximately three breaths in this amount of time, but this is a sufficient starting point for incorporating brief moments of total body relaxation into your day.

Make Breath Breaks a habit. After a few days of using the alarm, you will develop a sense of when one to two hours has lapsed. Begin to use this "internal alarm clock" rather than the physical alarm (watch or timer), and take your Breath Breaks whenever needed. When you master this technique, you will not need to pause what you are doing – you can continue walking, gardening, working, shopping, or cooking and still experience a quiet, mindful moment.

While working at the computer, I often find myself holding my breath and tensing my shoulders as tasks add up, words pour out, and opportunities for further connection, reading, and research multiply. Although Breath Breaks have become a habit, I'm human…and sometimes I need a reminder. Recently, I wrote a sticky note with the word: "BREATHE." I stuck this note to my computer, and now every time it catches my attention, I take a 30 second Breath Break. It grounds me and brings me back to the present moment…back to my breath…back to life.

Fun Tidbit: Did you know that proper breathing might actually help you LOSE WEIGHT? Worry and anxiety – which most of us do and have – generate a stress response. Prolonged stress releases excess cortisol and insulin. This can contribute to weight gain, especially in the abdominal region, and decreases your calorie-burning capacity. Don't dismiss Core Breathing as a waste of time. We know that deep breathing can decrease anxiety, so if you're interested in dropping a few pounds, you can consider it to be a calorie-burning activity!

Furthermore, breathing also promotes full digestive power. Think of metabolism as a fire in your body. What does a fire need to burn? Oxygen! Your body needs plenty of oxygen in order to maximize metabolic potential...to maximize calorie burning and fat-burning potential.

As Marc David (author of *The Slow Down Diet*) states, "The more we breathe, the more we digest, assimilate, and calorie burn."[42] If chewing fully is what STARTS the digestive process, BREATHING is what fuels the digestive process. During your next meal, take several deep, full, relaxed breaths. It's amazing what a difference it can make.

MINDFULNESS AND MEDITATION

So much has been written about the subjects of mindfulness and meditation that I can't even begin to scratch the surface here. However, I would be remiss to not at least mention the big M's while we're on the subject of rest, relaxation, and living in the moment.

Think of your body as a temple, your mind as the chatter of the devotees, and your soul as the altar – the most sacred space in the temple. When it comes to health and wellness, your body doesn't always know what it needs. Sure, it will give you cues, but you can't really hear those cues until you clear out the chatter (clear the mind) and spend some time in peace, worshipping at the altar. Only then can you clearly hear your soul.

"True silence is the rest of the mind; it is to the spirit what sleep is to the body, nourishment and refreshment."
–William Penn

This is why a daily practice of mindfulness and/or meditation is so important. These practices slow your mind and bring you into the moment, bringing you out of your "head" and into your heart. Both mindfulness (a state of active, open attention to the present) and meditation (intended to focus and quiet your mind) provide a direct connection – or link – between you body and your soul.

These practices are associated with Buddhist teachings, but they are completely nondenominational and can be practiced by anyone, at any time. You don't need to be sitting on a cushion with your legs crossed and incense wafting; you can meditate while walking, doing the dishes, or standing in line at the grocery store. Some people achieve a meditative state when they're dancing or exercising. The key is to seize multiple small opportunities during the day to calm your mind (meditate) and/or focus your attention on the present moment (mindfulness). Just like Core Breathing and taking regular Breath Breaks, these little moments add up and can work wonders when it comes to maintaining balance and sanity.

YIN AND YANG – FINDING ENERGETIC BALANCE

We touched upon the concept of energy in the "Womb Power" section of Chapter 5, but it's worth another look. Balancing your core energy fields can reshape your health and your life, and might even be the hidden key to feeling your best, especially if you feel "stuck" or like you've hit a plateau in your weight and/or health goals.

Newton's third law states that for every action, there is an equal and opposite reaction. One cannot exist without the other... This is the duality of the Universe. This "duality" also applies to the Taoist concept of Yin and Yang: two opposing (but complementary) energetic forces that are inherent in all living things. When the two halves (Yin and Yang) combine, they create wholeness.

It is important to note that nothing is completely Yin or completely Yang, and also that the nature of Yin and Yang flows and changes with time. As one aspect increases, the other decreases to maintain overall balance of the whole.[53]

Traditionally, Yin energy refers to the feminine energy that is in ALL individuals, even men. It is synonymous with being, receiving, resting, creating, and growing. Yang energy refers to the masculine energy that is in ALL individuals, even women. It is synonymous with fire, doing, conquering, and achieving. We need both Yin and Yang energy to survive and to thrive. **One is not "better" than the other; the key is to find balance and harmony between them, because when these two opposing forces are not in harmony, discord results.**

We live in a world that favors an out-of-balance masculine/Yang model for everyone, women included. Lack of time in nature, overscheduled, over-busy lives, becoming out of touch with our menstrual cycles and the ebb and flow of energy that goes with them – all of these modern afflictions can influence our health and our happiness.

Personally, I suffer from excess Yang and must consciously tend to my Yin energy. Here's a quick story from my own life. A few years ago, I consulted with Kim, a Tibetan medicine practitioner, about irregular menstrual cycles, pain on the right side of my body, and dermatological issues (acne and psoriasis) on the right side of my body. Kim discovered that my left (Yin) side was completely stagnant and felt blocked. My right (Yang) side was energetically dominant. As described above, Yin energy is grounded, nurturing, restful, and focused on receiving and "being." Yang energy is fiery, ambitious, highly structured (sometimes even a bit rigid), and focused on "doing" and "going." Guess which is a perfect description of me? You got it. Yang.

Although outwardly I looked feminine, my energy – my life force (my prana, my chi) – was highly masculine! Kim determined that my long-standing energy imbalance had created toxicity in the right side of my body, hence the pain, skin issues, and menstrual irregularity.

My feminine energy was blocked, and my masculine energy was sick and tired! As stated on www.dailyom.com:

"Maintaining harmony between the left side and the right side, the feminine and masculine, is a key to wholeness... We can foster awareness of our own

relative state of balance by tuning in to our bodies. When you close your eyes and scan your body, what do you see? You may find that most of your ailments, from acne to muscle tension, occur on the left side of your body. This might indicate that your feminine aspect is out of balance in some way. Similarly, if you notice a lot of tension in your right shoulder, perhaps your masculine side is overtaxed or weakened. Just noticing an imbalance is the beginning of healing it."[54]

Check in with yourself... How does this information strike you? Are you open to it? Do you sense an energetic imbalance in your own body?

Women's health practitioner Tami Kent feels that we – as women – must define new holistic measures of success in order to maintain our Yin energy in today's Yang world. Kent is hopeful that we can achieve this balance by tuning into our bodies and our intuition on a regular basis. She states, "Taking breaks from your schedule, seeing an illness as an opportunity for retreat, or stepping out of roles at work or home that no longer satisfy you can make space to fundamentally change the way you are inhabiting your days. As more feminine energy is reclaimed – and with it, the connection to our inner fire – the masculine structures will transform."[3]

EXERCISE – Check Your Yin:

Consider the following questions to determine whether (or not) you're taking the appropriate steps to nurture and maintain your Yin energy:

How am I sharing my gifts, talents, and time with the world? In turn, how am I accepting support from the world and people around me?

When was the last time I received massage or any other form of touch (sensual or otherwise)?

Am I on a team (receiving support), or am I "driving" my life alone?

Am I resting and enjoying myself proportionately to the amount of time and energy I spend accomplishing tasks that feel difficult and/or draining?

Have I spent time with my female friends lately?

Have I spent any time in unhurried, unrushed stillness?

What have I done to take care of – or beautify – my body? How about my home?

Am I in touch with my dreams? Do I remember them in the morning?

Am I tending to, growing, nurturing, or caring for anything or anyone (i.e. a garden, a pet, or a loved one)? If so, am I doing so out of obligation or because I want to?

Have I spent enough time in nature? When was the last time I actually touched the earth?

When was the last time I noticed the moon or gazed at the night sky?

When was the last time I did something creative? When was the last time I felt connected, alive, and in a state of "flow?"

When was the last time I danced or moved my body in a freely expressive way?

If you could use a bit more energetic balance in your life – especially if you're a bit too Yang – let me suggest the following technique.

EXERCISE – Find Energetic Balance:

Sit cross-legged on the floor (or ultimately, sit outside on the ground).

Begin with alternate nostril breathing, a breathing technique (or pranayama) from the yogic tradition that helps to calm and center the mind. Because it helps harmonize the right and left hemispheres of the brain and balance the "nadis" (energy channels that run through the body), it is an excellent way to prepare for the rest of this balancing exercise.

To do alternate nostril breathing:

- *Press your right thumb into your right nostril (to compress it) and inhale gently through your left nostril.*

- *Pause for a moment, and then close your left nostril with your right ring (fourth) finger. Release thumb from right nostril. Exhale through the right nostril.*

- *Pause for a moment. Now inhale through your right nostril, keeping your ring finger on the left nostril. When you reach the "top" of your inhalation, pause briefly, compress your right nostril with your thumb, and release your ring finger from your left nostril. Exhale gently through your left nostril.*

- *That was one round.*

- *Continue to breathe in through one side and out through the other. To walk you through another round, inhale through the left nostril, compress the left nostril, and then release the right nostril. Exhale through the right nostril, inhale through the right nostril, and then compress the right nostril and release the left nostril. Exhale through the left. Again... In through the left, out through the right, in through the right, out through the left.*

- Complete up to 9 rounds of alternate nostril breathing, ending with an exhalation on the left. Keep your eyes closed and your breathing relaxed and easy. Never, ever force.

- NOTE: Stop if you feel dizzy or lightheaded. Avoid this exercise if you have high blood pressure or any breathing difficulties such as asthma. Practicing on an empty stomach is preferred.

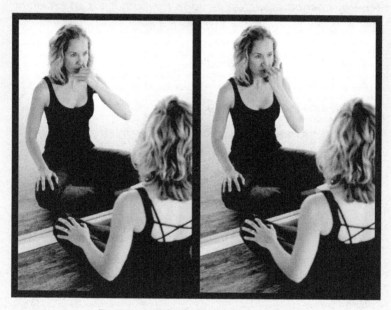

Finger position for alternate nostril breathing

After 9 rounds of alternate nostril breathing, bring your right hand to the center of your chest, bringing your masculine "doing" energy to your heart and solar plexus chakras (chakras are focal points, or loci, of energy). This simple action of placing your right hand over your heart energizes your centers of love, connection, self-esteem, and sense of self.

Place your left hand on the ground, palm down. This roots your feminine "being" energy, and literally "grounds" you, *allowing you to receive the present moment.*

If it feels awkward to place your hand flat on the ground, place your hand – palm down – on your left thigh.

Remain in this position, breathing deeply and easily, for 2-3 minutes. Your eyes can be closed or gently open during this portion of the exercise.

During your last few breaths, bring your left hand off the ground (or thigh) and place it over your right hand so that both hands are crossed over your heart. Hold your hands over your heart, breathing deeply into the present moment.

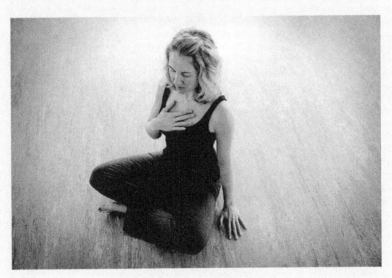

Hand placement for 2-3 minute meditation

"No one saves us but ourselves.
No one can and no one may.
We ourselves must walk the path."
–Buddha

Chapter 12

MOVE MORE

INCIDENTAL MOVEMENT

You can spot-train your core all day long, but the key to letting those strong, toned muscles shine through is to move more throughout the day, every day. The healthiest, longest-living people in the world aren't those who train hard once per day at the gym and then go home (or to the office) and sit; rather, longer lives and better health are found in people who move often, at fairly easygoing paces, throughout the day.

Did you know that each hour you spend sitting in front of the television after age 25 may shave 21.8 minutes off your life expectancy?[55] In another recent study, every two hour increase in sitting time was related to a 6% increased risk of lung cancer, an 8% increased risk of colon cancer, and a 10% increased risk of endometrial cancer.[56]

Although sitting periodically is, of course, fine, and standing all day long would create its own set of overuse issues and injuries, it is absolutely true that modern society SITS TOO MUCH.

"Incidental movement" is one of the top habits of healthy people regardless of age or stage of life. Incidental movement includes any activity built up in small amounts over the day; for example, walking up and down the stairs, or walking to and from your car. Incidental movement can prevent back pain, contribute to healthy aging, and can even make you more productive at home and at work. There's nothing more mind numbing (and creativity-depleting) than sitting for hours at a time without moving your body.

For me, incidental movement includes my twice-daily walks to and from my son's bus stop for drop-off and pick-up, alternating between sitting on a stool and standing at my stand-up desk while working, standing or pacing when I talk on the phone, and actively seeking parking spots that are the farthest away from the store. I also look at (formerly dreaded) tasks such as laundry and emptying the dishwasher as ways to burn a few extra calories AND fit more natural movements – squatting, bending, lifting, loading, and carrying – into my day.

One fun way to train yourself to move more is to attach a quick movement routine to something you already do every day. I have heard this referred to as "habit stacking," or using the power of "anchor habits." Whatever you want to call it, the basic idea is to build new habits by taking advantage of old habits that are already hardwired into your brain. Start simple; harness the positive snowball effect (small victories adding up)! One example is to do 10 countertop pushups every morning as you brew your coffee. Or try my bathroom fitness routine, which includes 10 squats, 10 countertop pushups, and 10 triceps dips every time you use the restroom. That's easily 4-5 times per day, so that's 40-50 additional squats, pushups, and triceps dips each day.

You can also enact the 30-30 Rule, which we covered in Chapter 9. This is especially great if you have a desk job. Every 30 minutes, or perhaps every time you shift to a new project or task, take 30 seconds to stand up and move. The simple act of rising from your chair to stand up and stretch or shake out your arms and legs will get your blood flowing from your feet to your head, thereby improving circulation and reducing the risk of blood clots and swelling in the lower extremities.

Movement is truly lifesaving, and "incidental movement" is just as important as getting your 30-45 minutes of formal "exercise" each day!

"If I am conscious of incidental movement, does that mean I don't have to exercise?"

No. In addition to moving more throughout the day, it is important to also establish a regular fitness routine. But here's the key – you have to enjoy it. Exercise is NOT punishment...nor is it something you should do just to work off the cheeseburger you ate. In order to make ANY new habit a habit that lasts, you must find the joy in it. My friend Yvette calls this "soul soaring fitness," which I think is absolutely beautiful.

Did you know that endorphins – "endogenous morphine" or feel-good, pain-relieving neurotransmitters – are emitted during meditation, exercise, and sex? As I always say, "It's not a good day if I don't sweat at least once!"

Use this as impetus to explore the world of fitness. Find something active that you love, and then do it consistently. Whether it's walking, tennis, golf, swimming, ice-skating, cycling, step aerobics, Zumba® classes, or a fitness video at home...it doesn't matter. Everyone's tastes are different, so explore and see what best suits YOU. **Fall in love with movement and you'll never have to "exercise" another day in your life!**

> **"Fitness doesn't have to be a duty. It doesn't have to mean charts and graphs and heart rate printouts. It should be a pleasurable part of your life, and it should include things that you do purely because you enjoy them. Fun is an ingredient that people often forget in their fitness program."**
> **–Laird Hamilton**

A FEMININE PERSPECTIVE ON FITNESS

Imagine a mash-up of traditional therapeutic exercises – squats, bridges, bird-dogs, and kegels – combined with hip circles, bust slides, booty pops, and shimmies. That's FemFusion® Fitness! We combine the health benefits of therapeutic exercise with the fun of a group fitness class. As participant Erin states:

"I have low back issues and have been essentially pain free so long as I do my one FemFusion class a week. I actually think the FemFusion classes are, for me, more valuable than going to a physiotherapist or chiropractor and, as an added bonus, I get a killer workout and have much more fun!"

This is not a plug for my program; rather, it's a testament to the power of moving your body in all directions and finding something that's fun and exciting for YOU. For many women, this means getting out of the rut of straight-plane linear movement, and freeing themselves from the bonds of "regular" (i.e. gym-based, or treadmill-based) exercise that can feel boring or lackluster. **If you want to feel good, move in a way that makes you HAPPY.**

When you start exercising in a way that fits your body and your personality, you will feel better and stronger both physically and emotionally, and that's a very empowering thing.

> **"Exercise because you love your body,**
> **not because you hate it."**
> **–Author Unknown**

I asked several women to tell me what they look for in a fitness routine. The following is a sample of their responses.

Anna, 40:
"In high school and college I wanted to run and play like the boys – I didn't really realize that there was a feminine quality underneath it all, waiting to come out. I just wanted to be able to sink as many free throws as them, I wanted to steal home base, and I wanted to slam my racquet just as hard – if not harder – than they did. But as I've gotten older, I've really come to appreciate the sexuality of being a woman and the way movement makes me feel connected with my body. I still love tennis and more 'hardcore' sports but I also appreciate more feminine forms of movement. I love dance, and I love feeling like I can shape and tone my body to look my best. So now I love movement for the intrinsic reason of feeling sexy and strong, but for extrinsic reasons too. I've got to admit, it's nice when other people notice and appreciate the beauty of me-in-motion. But mostly, I simply love the way I feel when I'm moving beautifully."

Sara, 35:
"I like to sweat, and I need variety. Whatever I do, it has to be high energy and upbeat."

Shanda 27:
"I do not like group exercise – it's intimidating. I'm a solo exerciser."

Jen, 34:
"I like having a partner to help motivate and encourage me."

There are as many different opinions about exercise as there are women in this world. Every female has her own priorities, goals, and desires when it comes to fitness, so I certainly can't expect every woman to be a great "fit" for the *Lady Bits* program without allowing some room for individuality.

Lady Bits encourages regular participation in fitness activities in addition to the Inner Core Energizer routine. I call these fitness activities **Sustained Physical Movement (SPM)**. SPM activities do not need to be part of a formal exercise program; you do not need to join a gym or purchase new gear. The key is to **move your body** at a level that elevates your heart rate and activates all of the major muscle groups for at least 30 minutes, five times per week. You don't even have to call it "exercise" if that word intimidates you or otherwise turns you off – SPM is simply "movement," and it's meant to feel GOOD.

I developed the fitness portion of the *Lady Bits* program to be a well-rounded exercise plan that strengthens and tones the entire body. Whereas the Inner Core Energizer focuses primarily on the core, the additional SPM activities are important for total-body conditioning.

I have been a part of the physical therapy and fitness worlds long enough to realize that attention spans are relatively short and that interests rapidly shift and change. Fitness trends come and go, and people enjoy sampling new things. No problem! As long as you consistently complete the Inner Core Energizer three times per week, you may supplement with whatever SPM activities you wish.

I want to keep you interested for the long haul, because **fitness is a long-term investment**. It takes time to see results, and in order to maintain the results, you must continue to invest time and effort with a consistent fitness routine. The great news is that it is absolutely worth it.

SUSTAINED PHYSICAL MOVEMENT (SPM) EXAMPLES

The following are some examples of SPM activities. Pick one or two that sound the most appealing and realistic for you, and do not be afraid to change activities when you need to freshen up your regimen.

If you're new to fitness training, be sure to start slow and don't judge yourself. You're getting out there and moving your body, and that's what matters.

WALKING

Consider this: A walk a day may keep premature death away. A recent large-scale study found that movement and activity makes a difference in your health, even if you are not at your ideal weight.[57]

Scientists looked at the effects of obesity and exercise on 334,161 European men and women over the course of 12 years. They found that people who engaged in moderate levels of daily exercise – equivalent to an energetic 20-minute walk – were 16% to 30% less likely to die than those classified as inactive.[57]

Although the impact of exercise was greatest among people at an ideal weight for their height/body type, those with a high body mass index (BMI) saw a benefit, as well. In an interview for *The Guardian*, one of the study's co-authors – Professor Nick Wareham – stated: "Helping people to lose weight can be a real challenge and, whilst we should continue to aim at reducing population levels of obesity, public health interventions that encourage people to make **small but achievable changes in physical activity** can have significant health benefits and may be easier to achieve and maintain."[58]

Walking is one of the most fundamental – and also one of the best – total body conditioning exercises. It is a natural strengthener for the inner core as well as the feet, legs, and hips. Although you may think of walking as a basic, linear (straight ahead) motion, there is actually an incredible amount of muscular activity and movement that takes place at the hips, knees, and ankles as you propel yourself along. Every time you take a step forward and place your foot, you use the muscles that internally and externally rotate your hips. You use your hip abductors every time you place your weight on one leg and swing the other leg forward. Your hamstrings contract as your leg swings through, and your tibialis anterior (shin) muscles activate to slow the forward motion so that you don't fall on your face. When dissected into its many phases, walking is a seriously complex motion!

Bringing it back to the inner core, the deep abdominal and back muscles are constantly "on" while walking in order to help you keep the trunk upright and stable. Furthermore, activation of the hip muscles naturally stimulates the pelvic floor. Janet Hulme, a physical therapist and researcher, has contributed a large body of evidence that documents the contributions of the hip rotator and adductor muscles to pelvic floor activation.[59] Many muscles are involved in walking, yet it is low impact, inexpensive (free, except for a good pair of shoes), and relaxing.

If you do not enjoy walking or don't have access to a safe walking environment, feel free to try another low-impact, rhythmic activity that contributes to total-body conditioning and improved cardiovascular fitness. Examples include biking (stationary or outdoor), elliptical training, cross-country skiing (simulated or outdoor), swimming, or rowing.

"What do you think about the 'barefoot shoes' that have become so popular?"

In the past, I encouraged my clients and friends to shop at athletic shoe retailers that specialize in analyzing gait mechanics. These retailers fit customers with shoes specific to their biomechanical needs, often placing people in stability or motion control shoes. Stability shoes can substantially lessen or even eliminate foot, knee, hip, or back pain since they help control excessive motion at the foot and ankle. This is a wonderful thing; however, I have come to question the value of stability shoes as I increasingly support the minimalist footwear movement.

Minimalist (or "barefoot") footwear provides little to no stability or motion control. The primary purpose of minimalist shoes is to provide some traction and to act as protection so that you do not cut your foot on a twig or shard of glass when enjoying the great outdoors.

Unlike stability shoes, minimalist shoes do not act as a crutch to control (or compensate for) biomechanical deficiencies; rather, the user is responsible for correcting their own biomechanical deficiencies. Wearing barefoot shoes requires that the user essentially re-learn how to walk in order to improve sensory awareness of the feet and ankles and strengthen muscles that have been previously underutilized. The aim of these shoes is to promote better foot mechanics naturally and intrinsically.

While barefoot shoes are not for everybody – for example, people who severely overpronate (a gait pattern in which the arches of the feet collapse inward) may not be able to transition to minimalist footwear without discomfort and possible injury – I think they are worthwhile for individuals who have a biomechanically "neutral" gait pattern. If you try barefoot shoes, understand that they are not for all occasions (sometimes you need more support or control), know that you'll have to build up to longer sessions of use, and always – I repeat, ALWAYS – listen to your body. They are not appropriate for all people. That being said, I regularly wear barefoot shoes and find that I use my leg and foot muscles more wholly than ever before.

INTERVAL TRAINING

Interval training is one of the best ways to amp up your metabolism, speed weight loss, and enhance total body conditioning. Interval training is defined as bouts of high intensity exercise followed by periods of lower intensity exercise or rest. There are a variety of interval training programs and describing them would be well beyond the scope of this book, so I recommend that you research interval training and hire a fitness professional to help design the most appropriate plan for you. It can be completely cardio-based (for example, intervals of two minutes of fast-paced walking followed by one minute of slower-paced walking for 30 minutes total), or it can involve resistance (weight) training. Resistance training is particularly important for women as it can help increase bone density and reduce the risk of osteoporosis.

> **Fun Tidbit:** Ladies, do not shy away from weight training. It will not bulk you up; rather, it will likely slim you down due to the metabolism-boosting effects of increasing lean muscle mass. More importantly, weight training is protective against the natural age-related decline in muscular strength and bone and muscle mass. Just remember to "zip up," exhale on exertion, and be careful! Find a qualified fitness trainer who can help you get started.

For my personal interval training routine, I follow a plan adapted from Jade and Keoni Teta's book, *The Metabolic Effect Diet.* The Teta brothers are naturopathic doctors and certified sports and conditioning specialists. They describe Rest Based Training (RBT), which is a form of interval training that includes bouts of high intensity exercise followed by periods of rest. With RBT you move from one high intensity exercise to the next without taking prescribed rest breaks; rather, **you rest only when needed**. When you rest, you do so for as long as necessary in order to fully recover. The theory is that one-size-fits-all interval training routines with mandatory rest breaks after each round of intense exercise may cause you to pace yourself and will prevent you from achieving the intensity of exercise needed to amp up your metabolic rate. The Teta brothers state that you should, "push hard, rest hard and then do it again."[60]

A word of caution if you have – or think you have – adrenal fatigue: high intensity interval training might be too much of a stressor at this time in your life, and it could actually be contributing to your condition.

Here's a good rule of thumb for exercise: in general, exercise should always make you feel BETTER when you're done, not worse. It might feel hard when you're doing it, but you should feel revived and energized after... not wiped out for hours or for days. If you're dragging every day, if you have to force yourself to the gym, if you're experiencing injuries after your training sessions, if you're holding onto stubborn weight despite daily exercise...then you might need to rethink your fitness program and try something new. This is often something "easier" or LESS intense, which sounds counterintuitive when you're trying to get fit and healthy, but often it works. **Go with what your body NEEDS...not what you think it should need, or what your husband needs, or what your teenage daughter needs.** Honoring your body and following your internal wisdom will leave you feeling stronger, slimmer, and more energized.

One of my health coaching clients was terrified to let go of her daily hardcore sweat sessions when I encouraged her to tone it down to daily walking and focused core strengthening due to some health challenges she was experiencing. When she took my advice, she realized that she loved it. Although she's no longer the "cardio queen," she's still active, slim, and sleek. Most importantly, her new routine is more appropriate for her body's changing needs.

YOGA

My yoga teacher once said "You're only as healthy as your spine," and I couldn't agree more. Counting your sacral and coccygeal (tailbone) vertebrae, the vertebral column has 33 segments, each with joints above and below. Most of the vertebrae have joints off to the sides (facet joints) as well. The spine has the extremely important job of protecting your spinal cord – a column of nerves that connects your brain to the rest of your body. The spinal cord branches off into 31 pairs of nerve roots, each of which exit the spine through small openings on each side of the vertebrae. The spine has so many moving parts, and so many nerves moving through it, that it's essential to keep it strong, flexible, and moving freely. Yoga is a wonderful way to do just that. From Hatha to Kundalini to Ashtanga to Yin, there is a style of yoga to suit every fitness level and preference.

Yoga is a beautiful practice that (can be) one heck of a workout. If you have ever doubted that yoga can make you sweat, try a power yoga or Ashtanga class! Your heart rate will elevate as you lengthen and strengthen your muscles, your circulation will improve, and your body will become sculpted and strong. Personal appearance and fitness gains aside, after I became familiar with the Ashtanga sequence, I developed a sense of inner strength combined with a sublime feeling of calm as I mastered the art of lithely moving from one challenging pose to the next.

I recommend seeking out a beginner-level class, or taking some basic yoga classes before sampling a power yoga or Ashtanga class. If you'd rather practice at home, the website www.bemoreyogic.com is a free online yoga resource that I personally use and enjoy.

DANCE

By far, my favorite SPM activity is dance. Dance connects you to your body like no other form of movement. It is an amazing core strengthener, improves balance, allows you to express and feel your femininity, and fuses power with grace. Every form of dance utilizes the core muscles to help stabilize the trunk against your moving arms and legs. Your core, including your deep inner core, is active the entire time you are on the dance floor; if it were not, you would lose your footing and fall flat.

Bellydance in particular is art in motion. It is a fun, low-impact cardiovascular workout, a powerful inner core strengthener, and tailor-made for a woman's body. The origins of this ancient dance are vague, but a leading theory is that bellydance was a dance performed by women, for women (and not intended for male entertainment). Grandmothers and mothers taught their granddaughters and daughters bellydance as a way to isolate and strengthen the muscles that are used during childbirth. Knowing how to move the pelvis, connecting with the pelvic floor, and strengthening the deep abdominals are essential for the pushing phase of labor – of course our predecessors understood this!

The pelvic motions found in bellydance require focus and control, especially when the movements are small and isolated. Take a bellydance class or follow an instructional video; you'll be glad you did, and you'll probably be sore – in a good way – the next day.

Bellydance isn't your thing? Try Latin dance, country line dancing, or even pole dancing. Dance is also integrated into FemFusion® classes, if classes are offered in your area. My tagline is "move like a lady," and dance is such a beautiful (and fun) way to tap into your inner goddess.

As Sheila Kelley, founder of S Factor™ Fitness (a dance-based workout) said in her 2012 TEDx talk, "Step into the grandeur, the beauty, the gorgeousness, the sway, the curve, the power, the FIRE of your body... I want you to go out and THROW A HIP CIRCLE in the middle of the Ralph's grocery store – just for the fun of it!"[61]

Dance can help you own and embody your innate inner goddess. When you let loose and unapologetically move your body the way it was meant to move, without self-imposed restriction or fear of judgment (from yourself or others), you will be amazed at how sexy, free, and alive you can feel.

JOGGING/RUNNING

For the purpose of the *Lady Bits* program, I do not recommend that you take up jogging unless you are already an avid runner and adore it – mind, body, and spirit. **If you love running, by all means…keep it up. But if you don't adore it, don't do it.** Contrary to popular belief, you don't have to run to be healthy.

Participating in lengthy sessions of high impact exercise such as long-distance running is tough on joints and can stress your pelvic floor, particularly if you have undergone surgery in the pelvic region, if you've recently given birth, or if – for any reason – you are recovering your pelvic floor strength. As mentioned in Chapter 9, the jarring effects of running and other high impact exercises can cause you to reach and exceed your "continence threshold" more quickly than lower impact fitness activities.[62] In other words, you may leak sooner if you are pounding pavement.

Need more evidence to support lower impact fitness options? As stated above, high impact activities are more likely to cause urinary incontinence. In addition to the hassle of cleaning up after an episode of incontinence, the embarrassment caused by urinary leakage can cause up to 20 percent of women to quit their fitness program.[62]

Beginning (and sticking to) a fitness regimen is difficult in its own right and excuses to quit abound. If you are just starting a regular fitness routine, maximize your chance of sticking with the program by choosing activities that will minimize discomfort and embarrassment. If you have any history of pelvic floor dysfunction or weakness, do yourself a favor and opt for something lower impact than running.

The focus of *Lady Bits* is being kind and gentle to the pelvic floor and core, and to your body as a whole. You certainly do not need to give up running if it is your favorite activity, but it is imperative to keep your pelvic floor muscles strong and supple, and to purchase quality footwear – whether it be traditional running shoes or "minimalist" footwear – from a reputable source.

HAVE FUN

> "People rarely succeed unless they have fun
> in what they are doing."
> –Dale Carnegie

Whatever you choose for your SPM sessions, from hiking to rowing to pole dancing, **remember to have fun!** Nothing is sexy about dragging yourself to the gym to do something you hate, so if you are not happy with your activity selection, change it.

If you tried walking 30 minutes five days per week and hate it, go swimming! If you can't stand the aerobics class you sampled, call up your girlfriends and go dancing at the hottest nightclub in town. Clubs are not only for the twenty-something set; dancing at a nightclub is perhaps the sweatiest, sexiest workout available, and they are open to all card-carrying adults.

The point is to enjoy yourself so fitness becomes a **priority** and not an option that ends up on the back burner. In order to make the *Lady Bits* program work for you, fitness needs to become a part of your daily routine. There is no way around it...so have fun with it!

Chapter 13

THE INNER CORE ENERGIZER

I've alluded to the Inner Core Energizer throughout this book...
Now it's time to introduce the routine!

The Inner Core Energizer involves all of your core muscles,
strengthening, toning, and increasing coordination so that you will be
able to effectively utilize the inner core muscles when you need them
most. The exercises are feminine and just a little bit flirty; I take you out
of linear, straight-plane movement patterns and introduce fluid, circular
motions that strengthen and mobilize your hips and spine. In short,
you're going to "move like a lady." Enjoy the way this feminine, fluid
movement makes you feel in your body.

I will provide brief descriptions of the individual exercises in the
Inner Core Energizer below, but please note that I have created two
videos that anyone with an Internet connection can access, for FREE, at
www.femfusionfitness.com/energizer. The first (instructional) video
goes through the routine in its entirety, with more verbal explanation
and descriptions of modifications for beginners and for women with
diastasis recti. It also shows progressions if you need more of a challenge.
Start with this video. The second (flow) video goes through the routine
much faster, with no breaks between movements and only with the more
advanced versions shown. This video is intended for women who are
familiar and comfortable with the routine.

A NOTE FOR WOMEN WHO ARE PREGNANT: It is typically
recommended that you should not begin an exercise program in your 2nd
or 3rd trimester if you were previously sedentary. However, if you were
exercising before pregnancy, and if you have been consistently exercising
up until now, then most of the exercises in the Inner Core Energizer are

safe for women in early pregnancy (1st and 2nd trimesters). Watch for positional considerations (i.e. be mindful not to spend too much time on your back), and avoid anything that's painful or uncomfortable. Of course, it is important to check with your healthcare provider first. He or she can guide you based on your specific needs.

Also, remember that your best resource for keeping strong and supple pelvic floor and core muscles, preventing back pain, and keeping control of your bodily functions both during and after pregnancy is to **MOVE MORE throughout the day**, each and every day. That really is the key! So don't forget about "incidental movement" and your SPM activities.

A NOTE FOR WOMEN WHO ARE NEWLY POSTPARTUM: The general rule of thumb is to wait to resume exercise until six weeks after delivery. If you've had a C-section, you must wait until all incisions are healed and your abdominal region is pain free. If you have ANY questions or reservations, please check with your doctor or midwife.

A REMINDER FOR WOMEN WITH DIASTASIS RECTI: Watch for the notes specific to DR in the exercise descriptions below.

INNER CORE ENERGIZER

The following list of exercises is lengthy, but the routine is meant to flow from one move to the next without breaks. In total, when flowing through, the entire routine takes 25 minutes. You will need a yoga mat and a yoga block or small, firm pillow.

> **All exercises are described below, and selected exercises are pictured. For best results, I recommend viewing the digital workout online at *www.femfusionfitness.com/energizer*. Two video options are provided; the first with detailed instructions and modifications, and the second without significant verbal instructions or breaks.**

Here we go! The first five exercises are designed to get you "into" your body, and to wake up your deep inner core muscles. The remaining exercises activate your entire core, as well as your hips and thighs. Pay attention to the energetic (chakra) activation, as well.

PELVIC ROCKS: Lie on your back with your hips and knees bent. Gently rock your pelvis forward (anterior pelvic tilt), and back (posterior pelvic tilt). As you rock forward, inhale deeply and let your belly and lower ribs expand. As you rock back, gently pull in your abdominal muscles and feel your low back pressing into the ground. Rock back and forth, smoothly, for 30-60 seconds.

Pelvic rocks mobilize and lubricate the joints of the spine and hips, improve blood flow to the pelvic region, and are a fantastic way to combine deep breathing with pelvic floor muscle activation.

PELVIC BOUNCES: In the same position as above, lightly bounce your pelvis on the ground. This should be a gentle movement (not jarring), and can be taken as quickly – or as slowly – as is comfortable for you. Bounce gently for 30 seconds.

Pelvic bounces activate your first and second chakras, improve pelvic circulation, and heighten inner core awareness.

STIRRING THE POT: Still lying on your back, bring your legs off the ground and firmly hold onto your knees with your hands. Use your arms to move your legs in a circular motion. Draw your knees apart and then toward one another. Your legs should be relaxed – they are just along for the ride. "Stir the pot" 5 times in one direction, then 5 times in the opposite direction.

This is an excellent way to continue to relax, stretch, and increase circulation to the hips and pelvic floor. It also lubricates the hip joints.

OPEN LIKE A BOOK: Continue to hold onto your knees with your hands. Allow your body to roll to one side (knees together), and then lift your top knee off the bottom knee, and roll to the other side. Roll to each side 3-5 times.

This exercise massages your sacrum and low back, stretches the inner thigh and groin area, and activates the pelvic floor.

30-SECOND BREATH MEDITATION: Lie comfortably on your back, with your legs slightly apart and your hands placed lightly over your belly. Initiate Core Breathing (Chapter 11). Imagine a bright light, growing, expanding, and filling your lower abdomen and pelvis. Allow this light to overflow and expand into your thighs, hips, and posteriorly into your buttocks and low back. Breathe slowly, deeply, and gently for 30 seconds.

This brief meditation focuses your attention on your inner core muscles and your lower chakras: your "powerhouse" when it comes to creative and sexual energy. The breathing helps center and ground you, and enhances your mind-body connection. White or golden lights are common colors to visualize, but if you are familiar with the chakra system you might want to visualize red and/or orange light. These are the colors associated with the root and sacral – the first and second – chakras.

REMINDER: View the digital workout online at www.femfusionfitness.com/energizer.

BRIDGE WITH BLOCK, INTO DEEP ABDOMINAL WAKE-UP: Lie on your back with your knees bent. Place a firm pillow, small fitness ball, or a yoga block between your knees. Engage your pelvic floor muscles and then tighten your buttocks. Roll up, one vertebra at a time, into a "bridge" position. Hold for 10 seconds. Avoid holding your breath!

Keeping your pelvic floor and buttocks engaged, roll down one vertebra at a time. Once your tailbone touches the ground, completely relax. Let your knees drop apart (remove the block) and breathe deeply. Repeat this sequence 2 more times.

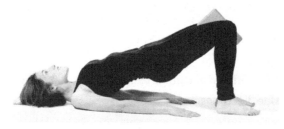

Bridge

Lady Bits

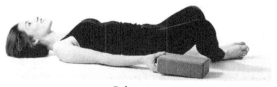

Relaxation

The final time, do not let your knees drop apart. Keep the block between your knees. Strongly engage your inner core muscles (pull the lowest band of abdominal muscles gently toward your spine) and use your abs and hip flexors to lift your knees toward your chest, and then to set your feet gently back onto the floor. Exhale as you lift your knees toward your chest, and inhale as you return your feet to the floor. Do not let your low back arch. Lift and lower your legs (keeping the block between your knees) 10 times.

The bridge portion of this series strengthens the inner core, buttocks, and hamstrings, and improves awareness of inner core contraction versus relaxation.

The leg lift portion of this series "wakes up" your deep abdominal muscles (and your hip flexors), preparing your muscles for the exercises ahead.

LONG LEG STRETCH: Lie on your side with your bottom leg bent for stability and your head propped on your hand if desired. Inhale as you lift your top knee toward your shoulder. Hold the back of your calf or thigh and stretch your leg up toward the ceiling as you exhale. Sweep your straight leg forward and down toward the floor as you inhale. As you exhale, bend your knee and sweep your leg up toward the ceiling once again. Sweep your leg around (and stretch your leg toward the ceiling) 5 times. Use your hands to push yourself up, swing yourself around, and switch sides. Repeat 5 times with the opposite leg.

This exercise – inspired by the "Side Leg Peel" in Sheila Kelley's S Factor™ workout – is not only sexy, it's also a fantastic stretch for the hamstrings and lubricates the hip joints.[63]

V-LEGS: Lie on your back with your knees bent. Find neutral spine position and strongly engage your deep abdominals. Bring both legs off the floor and straighten them toward the ceiling. Point your toes to activate the muscles in the back of your legs. Simply keeping your knees straight throughout this exercise will activate the muscles in the front of your legs. Open your legs into a "V" position, and then bring your legs together crossing your right leg over your left. Open your legs into a "V" again, then bring your legs together crossing your left leg over your right. You just completed one repetition.

Continue the exercise, alternating the leg cross. Inhale as the legs move apart, and exhale as they press together. Complete 10 repetitions (10 crosses of each leg).

V-Legs strengthens your deep abdominals, hip flexors, and hip adductors (inner thigh muscles). Strongly draw the legs together and slowly draw the legs apart to increase the challenge.

BUTTERFLY BRIDGE: Lie on your back with your knees bent. Let your knees fall apart. Tighten your buttocks. As you exhale, lift your hips off the floor and bring your knees together. As you inhale, return your hips to the floor and draw your knees apart. Keep your core muscles engaged throughout this exercise, and breathe steadily and smoothly. Feel the fire building in your lower chakras. Complete 10 repetitions.

This exercise strengthens your hip rotators, buttocks, pelvic floor, and hip adductors.

*PRANCE, INTO DEEP AB BLASTER: Lie on your back with your knees bent. Find neutral spine position and strongly engage your deep abdominals. Keep your deep abdominal muscles pulled in and maintain neutral spine position (don't let your back overly arch) as you bring both legs off the floor with your knees bent. Tap one foot to the floor, and then the other. This is one repetition of "Prance." Repeat 10 times.

For the "Deep Ab Blaster," continue to keep your abdominal muscles pulled in and maintain neutral spine position as you exhale and straighten your right leg. Pause, and inhale as you return it to the middle. Switch and exhale as you straighten your left leg. Pause, and inhale as you return it to the middle. You just completed one repetition. Complete 10 slow, controlled repetitions.

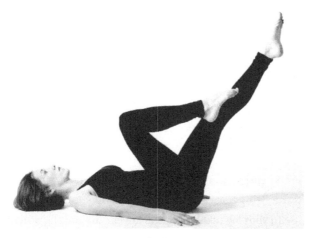

Deep Ab Blaster

For a "Deep Ab Blaster" challenge, place both hands on the thigh of your bent leg. Exhale as you press the thigh gently into the hands, and the hands gently into the thigh. Even though there's no movement, you will feel an increase in effort as you use your core to stabilize against the two opposing forces. Inhale as you switch sides. Exhale as you gently press your hands into the other thigh.

Remember to keep your abdominals pulled in and maintain neutral spine position throughout this series. Do not let your back overly arch. If you feel your back starting to arch off the ground, put your legs down, relax, and start over.

*Note for women with DR: Stick to the "Prance" portion of this series, using your hands to draw your rectus abdominis muscles together, toward the midline of our body. Zip up your core and do not let your low back arch. Remember to breathe steadily, with short, gentle exhalations each time you touch one foot to the floor during "Prance."

This exercise targets the transverse abdominis as well as the hip flexors. It's a great exercise for increasing core stability and awareness of how to find and maintain neutral spine position.

BRIDGE WITH HIP CIRCLES: Lie on your back with your knees bent. Engage your pelvic floor muscles and then tighten your buttocks. Roll up, one vertebra at a time, into a "bridge" position. Circle your hips 5 times one direction (like you're drawing a circle on the wall in front of you), and then reverse and circle your hips 5 times the other direction. Keep your hips/pelvis off the ground throughout, and breathe steadily.

This strengthens your hamstrings and buttocks, stretches the hip flexors, and lubricates the spine and hip joints.

SLALOM: Find neutral spine position and gently draw your abdominal muscles inward. Bring both legs off the floor and straighten them toward the ceiling. Bend your legs slightly at the knees. Lift your hips slightly off the floor as you twist your pelvis to strongly drive both knees to the right. Feel the left side of your abdominal muscles (your obliques) contracting. Now reverse and lift your hips slightly off the floor as you twist your pelvis to strongly drive both knees to the left. Feel the right side of your abdominal muscles (your obliques) contracting. You just completed one repetition.

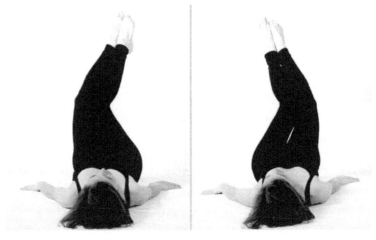

Slalom

Continue to twist your pelvis (lifting it slightly off the floor) with a focus on strongly driving your knees to the right and left. Complete 20 repetitions.

This is an intense abdominal strengthener meant to whittle the waistline and rid you of the dreaded "muffin top." It works your deep abdominal muscles with a focus on the internal and external obliques.

SUPERWOMAN WITH FOOT TAPS AND MINI REAR-LIFTS: Roll onto your stomach. Lengthen your spine and tighten your buttocks. Bring your upper body and both straight legs up off the floor and hold. Tap your feet together 10 times, and then relax your upper body and your legs back down to the ground. Follow with 3 "Mini Rear Lifts."

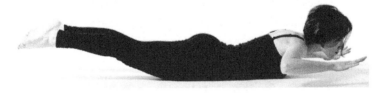

Superwoman

For Mini Rear Lifts: Keeping your upper body and your legs relaxed on the ground, **use your low back muscles** to lift your buttocks and pelvis up off the floor. Then press your pelvis down into the floor, lengthening your spine and tightening your buttocks. Repeat 3 times. Make the movement slow, small, and controlled with focused awareness. This is a very small movement (approximately one inch of motion), but it is an effective strengthener particularly for the erector spinae and multifidus muscles of the back.

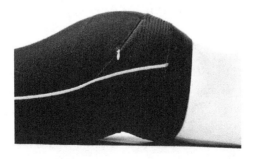

Mini Rear Lifts

Repeat "Superwoman + Foot Taps" followed by "Mini Rear Lifts" for a total of 3 repetitions of the entire sequence.

REMINDER: View the digital workout online at www.femfusionfitness.com/energizer.

CHILD'S POSE ALL DIRECTIONS: Sit back onto your heels with your arms stretched out in front of you and your chest low to the ground. Relax in this position for 15-20 seconds, breathing deeply. Without moving your feet or hips, walk your hands to the left, keeping your chest low to the ground. Feel a stretch in the right side of your trunk and hips as you relax in this position for 15-20 seconds, breathing deeply. Again, without moving your feet or hips, walk your hands to the right, keeping your chest low to the ground. Feel a stretch in the left side of your trunk and hips as you relax in this position for 15-20 seconds, breathing deeply. Return to the starting position and take another deep breath.

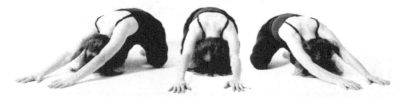

Child's Pose All Directions

This resting pose stretches and lengthens the hip and trunk muscles.

KNEELING FOOT/TOE STRETCH WITH HANDS CLASPED OVERHEAD: Start in child's pose. Dorsiflex at the ankles so that your toes are on the floor. Next, roll up into a kneeling position so that you're sitting on your heels with your toes on the floor. Feel a deep stretch in the bottom of your feet. Keep your feet and ankles parallel as you clasp your hands overhead, stretching and opening your shoulders, chest, and back. Breathe deeply and hold for 15-20 seconds. If your feet cramp at any time, relax your feet so that the tops of your feet rest on the floor.

This deeply stretches the knees, ankles, and the muscles of the toes and feet, preparing you for the deep squats that are ahead.

CHEST EXPANSION (FOR THE SOLAR PLEXUS): Still sitting on your heels, bring your hands down and grasp your heels firmly. Gently arch your back, opening your heart and your solar plexus (third) chakra. Imagine a ball of yellow light shining forward, flowing out of your body. Yellow is the color of your third chakra. Hold for 15-20 seconds, breathing deeply.

This continues to stretch the knees, ankles, and the muscles of the toes and feet, and begins to activate the middle (solar plexus and heart) chakras.

KUNDALINI HEART OPENER, INTO BUST CIRCLES: Still sitting on your heels, allow your feet to relax down so that the tops of your feet are on the ground. Lightly grasp your knees with your hands. Inhale as you arch your back, and then exhale as you round your back, grasping your knees gently throughout. Your mid-back should be the primary mover in this exercise. Arch and round your back 20 times, breathing with the movement and alternating fairly quickly between the two positions. If you wish, you can visualize green light shooting forward as you inhale and arch your back, and being contained within your heart as you exhale and round your back. Green is the color of the heart (fourth) chakra.

Still holding on lightly to your knees or thighs, circle your heart to the left 5 times, and then to the right 5 times, as if you're drawing a circle on the ground beneath you.

This lubricates the spine and activates the core muscles, fuses breath with movement, and continues to activate the middle (solar plexus and heart) chakras. Your energy should really be flowing now!

*NAUGHTY CAT, INTO ROCKING HORSE: Start on your hands and knees. Circle your pelvis as if you were drawing a circle on the wall behind you, and then allow your spine to move in a circle as well. Repeat 10 times in one direction, then reverse and switch directions.

Return to a neutral position on your hands and knees for "Rocking Horse." Draw your abdominals in (toward your spine) without tucking your tailbone under. Keeping your knee bent, bring your right leg behind you (toe pointing up toward the ceiling) as you inhale. As you exhale, bring your right knee toward your nose. You can round your back slightly as you do this. Repeat 10 times, and then switch sides. Be sure to re-set your core muscles between sides, if needed.

Note for women with DR: You can modify this exercise by placing your hands on a 2nd or 3rd stair (or something of that height) to reduce the downward pull of gravity on your strained abdominal fascia.

"Naughty Cat" is a flowing exercise that gently mobilizes the spine and takes you out of the linear/straight plane movement patterns to which most traditional exercises are confined. If you are not accustomed to making circular motions with your hips and pelvis, the pelvic circles might feel difficult and awkward at first. They will become easier with time – just keep practicing! Let your sexiest self shine through as you move through your full range of motion.

"Rocking Horse" strengthens the hips, buttocks, low back, and deep abdominals.

KNEELING SERIES (HIP PUMPS, CIRCLES, AND PELVIC LIFTS): Kneel on the floor with your hips and trunk straight (this position is called tall kneeling). Your knees should be no more than hip-width apart. Slowly lower yourself to sit back onto your heels. Now "zip up" (engage your pelvic floor and deep abdominals), tighten your buttocks, and exhale as you press your hips forward and up. Repeat 10 times.

Move into hip circles. Return to the tall kneeling position, knees no more than hip-width apart. Smoothly circle your hips to the left (move your hips forward, to the left, to the back, to the right, and then forward again). Complete 5 circles, then reverse and complete 5 circles to the right.

Now separate your knees are wider than shoulder-width apart, and lower your hips toward your heels. Imagine that you're lifting a silk handkerchief off the ground and pulling it into your body (do a kegel). Use your hips, thighs, and pelvic floor to lift your body a few inches up, and then lower yourself back down. After you lower yourself back down, relax the pelvic floor muscles, releasing the imaginary handkerchief. Repeat 5 times, slowly.

These are stellar moves to increase hip and pelvic mobility and pelvic floor strength. In addition, they are great gluteal, back, and thigh strengtheners.

SIDE PLANK WITH OBLIQUE TWISTS: Lie on your side, propped up on your elbow, legs stacked and your knees slightly bent for stability. Lift your bottom hip off the ground so that your body is in a straight line from your shoulders to your knees. Be sure that your elbow is directly under your shoulder. Reach your top arm up toward the ceiling, and then swoop it underneath your body as if you're reaching for something behind you. Hug your bellybutton to your spine and exhale as you twist and reach under. Inhale as you reach up toward the ceiling, keeping your hips elevated the entire time. Repeat 10 times. Return your hips to the floor, and then switch sides. Advanced practitioners can perform this exercise in a full side plank (with the feet staggered or stacked).

This waist-slimming exercise is a total core strengthener. It's also fantastic for the shoulders and upper back.

*PLANK WITH HIP-DROP: Roll onto your stomach. Bring your elbows directly under your shoulders. Strongly engage your abdominal muscles and lift your pelvis off the ground so that your body is in a straight line from your shoulders down to your knees. Advanced practitioners may lift the knees off the ground in order to "plank" from your elbows and toes. Beginner or advanced, be sure that your core muscles are strong and "set" and that your body is straight like a plank; do not let your low back round or sag.

Continue to keep your abdominals pulled in as you drop your hips a few inches down on the right. Swoop your pelvis up and over (as if you're moving over a barrel), and then drop your hips a few inches down on the left. Keep your feet together throughout this exercise, and breathe steadily, exhaling as you drop your hips. Repeat 10 hip drops on each side.

Note for women with DR: Stick to the beginner variation of "planking" from your elbows and knees. Consider modifying this exercise even further by placing your bent elbows on the 2nd or 3rd stair (or something of that height) to reduce the downward pull of gravity on your strained abdominal fascia. Remember to breathe steadily, with short, gentle exhalations each time you drop your hips.

Planks are fantastic total core strengtheners. This variation targets the abdominal obliques as well as the transverse abdominis and deep back muscles.

REMINDER: View the digital workout online at www.femfusionfitness.com/energizer.

DOWNWARD FACING DOG WITH ALTERNATING KNEE BENDS: From your plank position, tuck your toes under and exhale as you use your deep abdominal muscles to press up and back, lifting your bottom toward the ceiling. If you need a more gentle transition, take a break by moving through child's pose before going into the full "Downward Dog" position. When in "Downward Dog," keep your abdominals pulled in as you breathe steadily into your back ribs. Focus on lifting your tailbone up toward the ceiling and pressing your chest toward your thighs. Rhythmically bend one knee at a time, allowing your hips and pelvis to move naturally. Hold the position for 30 seconds, alternating knee bends and breathing steadily.

This rhythmic exercise stretches the hamstrings, low back, and buttocks.

PIGEON POSE: From "Downward Dog," bring your right knee forward toward your right wrist. Slowly inch your right shin and foot toward the midline of your body until your foot is directly below your left hip. Now straighten your left leg behind you. Feel the weight of your torso centered over your pelvis and lower both sides of your pelvis toward the floor. Your hips should be level. Make sure one side is not higher than the other; if necessary, place a folded blanket or yoga block under the right buttock so your pelvis isn't off kilter. Be meticulous about keeping your hips level in order to feel the full effects of the pose and to keep your lower back safely aligned. As your hips settle into the pose, press your fingertips firmly into the floor and lengthen your torso up toward the ceiling. See photo for reference. Hold for 30 to 60 seconds, and then switch sides.

This classic yoga pose is a hip opener that deeply stretches the hip rotators and hip flexors.

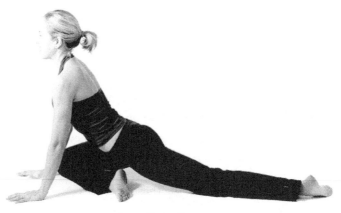

Pigeon Pose

DEEP SQUAT WITH KEGELS: Deeply squatting (sitting on your haunches) is a fantastic way to stretch and strengthen all of the muscles of the deep core and legs. It can also help relieve back pain since it strengthens the muscles in the lumbar region. Culturally, we have moved away from deeply squatting; however, it is one of the most natural human postures. For millions of years, before the invention of chairs and toilets, squatting was the way humans relaxed, toileted, and gave birth. An unfortunate consequence of our move away from squatting is a decrease in pelvic floor strength and flexibility as well as generalized tightening/stiffening of our lower extremity muscles and joints.

You might look at this exercise with horror, thinking "I can't do that!" Don't worry – you will get there! Squats are perfectly safe and achievable, even if it takes multiple sessions to increase your range of motion. There are a few pointers to remember no matter where you are in the progression described:

- First, your feet should be placed slightly wider than the pelvis. A foot placement that is too narrow or too wide will strain your knees.

- Second, your feet should point forward in order to maintain neutral alignment at the knees and hips.

- Third, the distance between your knees should not be significantly wider or narrower than the distance between your feet. Do not let your knees fall in, or "knock" together.

- Sit back and try to keep your shins as vertical to the floor as possible.

- Finally, remember to keep your heart lifted and your pelvis untucked the entire time.

At first, you may not be strong or flexible enough to lower yourself down into (or come up from) a deep squat. Work up to a full squat by following the progression below. It may take several weeks to move from level one to level three – that's fine! Take your time.

You should never feel pain when doing these exercises. A feeling of stretch is desirable, as is a feeling of muscle fatigue from working muscles you do not regularly use. **However, pain is not okay**. Back off by a level if you feel pain as you progress from level one through three. For example, if you feel pain when attempting level two, return to level one. Do not progress to level two until you can attempt it without pain.

An important note for people with hip and/or knee replacements: Do not attempt the squat progression if you are following post-surgical precautions. Even if you no longer have any surgical precautions, avoid the fully weight bearing squat (level three). Stick to level one, and possibly progress to level two if you have been through a full course of physical therapy and do not have any residual pain. Consult with your physician if you have any concerns.

Deep Squat Progression

Level One (not pictured): Sit on a chair with a firm seat, and elevate your feet on a stepstool. Keep your feet flat on the stepstool – not on your tiptoes! Your knees should be higher than your hips. Straighten and lengthen your back; do not round your back or let your tailbone tuck under. Feel as if someone is pulling a string in a diagonal line from your tailbone up through the top of your head toward the ceiling. Stay in this position for at least 30 seconds to stretch the ankles, knees, and hips, and to strengthen the muscles of the low back. Breathe deeply.

Level Two (see photo): Place a pillow or rolled yoga mat behind your knees, and stand with your heels on a rolled yoga mat or firm cushion.

Hold onto the back of a chair for support and slowly lower yourself down into a deep squat. Do not let your back round or your tailbone tuck under. Lengthen your spine and lift your heart, trying to maintain a neutral spine position. Stay in this position for at least 30 seconds to stretch the ankles, knees, and hips, and to strengthen the muscles of the low back. Breathe deeply.

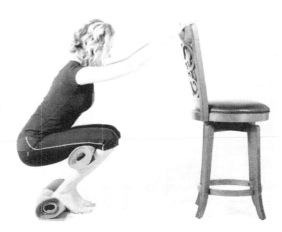

Squat Progression: Level Two

Level Three (see photo): Without holding onto a chair for support, slowly squat down and place your elbows on your knees. You may continue to use the rolled yoga mat behind your knees to take some pressure off the knee joints, or you may remove it for a deeper hip and thigh stretch. You may continue to use the rolled yoga mat or cushion under your heels, or you may remove it for a deeper ankle and calf stretch. Some people will be able to place their feet flat on the ground – that's wonderful! Do not let your back round or your tailbone tuck under. Lengthen your spine and lift your heart. Stay in this position for at least 30 seconds to stretch the ankles, knees, and hips, and to strengthen the muscles of the low back. Breathe deeply.

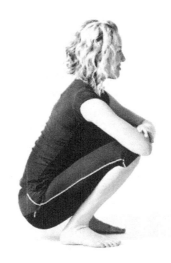

Squat Progression: Level Three

Deep Squat Progression: The Final Step

Add kegels. When you have found the squat position that works for you (level one, two, or three), bring your attention to your pelvic floor muscles. In a deep squat the pelvic floor muscles are slightly lengthened. Squatting is a fantastic position to really sense your pelvic floor muscle contraction and relaxation and a great position in which to practice doing kegels against gravity. Complete 5-10 kegels, remembering to fully relax between repetitions.

FROG SQUATS: From your deep squat position, bring your heels together, toes pointing outward. Your heels can be off the floor. Place your hands down on the ground in front of you. If your hamstrings are tight, place your hands on a yoga block or two. Exhale as you straighten your legs and reach your buttocks up toward the ceiling; your heels will come to the floor. Now inhale as you bend your knees deeply, returning to the starting position. If this breathing pattern doesn't feel good to you, listen to your intuition. You can also inhale as you straighten your legs and reach your buttocks toward the ceiling, and exhale as you bend your knees. In fact, this is the classic breathing technique for this exercise as practiced in Kundalini yoga. For this exercise in particular, go with what feels good in your body. Repeat 10 times.

This classic Kundalini exercise is a great strengthener for your hip adductors (inner thighs), pelvic floor, and buttocks. It also increases your heart rate, stretches your hamstrings, and moves energy throughout your entire body.

HIP ACTIVATOR SERIES: Lie on your back in a butterfly position, with the soles of your feet touching and your knees bent and dropped apart. Engage your pelvic floor and your deep abdominals, and then lift your hips/pelvis off the ground approximately 4-5 inches. Feel the activation in your outer hip and thigh muscles, as well as in your pelvic floor and groin region. Hold this position for two minutes. Yep, two minutes! Breathe steadily throughout, keeping your hips elevated the entire time. Your hip and thigh muscles might begin to quiver, and that's okay. Muscular fatigue is what we're hoping to achieve with this exercise. That being said, pain is never okay – certainly rest (or stop) if needed.

Throughout the two minutes, be sure that your lower back doesn't hurt or begin to arch. Keep you lower abdominals gently engaged, and think about lengthening your tailbone forward, toward the front of the room. Breathe steadily. If at any time you feel pinching or fatigue in the low back, take a break. When you begin again, lengthen your tailbone forward (thereby creating space in the spine) even more.

After two minutes have passed, with your hips still elevated and your core muscles still engaged, bring your knees up (i.e. closer together) 1-2 inches. Hold for 15 seconds, breathing steadily. Now bring your knees up another 1-2 inches and hold for 15 seconds. Finally, bring your knees up another 1-2 inches and hold for 15 seconds. As you move your knees up (closer together) your feet will move closer and closer to a flat-on-the-floor position. Recall that your hips are elevated the entire time, and you're breathing steadily throughout.

All together, the "Hip Activator Series" takes approximately 2 minutes, 45 seconds. When you're finished, return your hips to the floor and spend 15 seconds rocking your pelvis forward and back to release your core muscles. Breathe deeply and relax.

NOTE: If at any time this exercise feels like "too much," stop and lower your pelvis to the ground, straighten your legs, and gently shake them out. There is no need to push yourself too hard, before you're ready.

The "Hip Activator Series" brings heat and fire to the buttocks, pelvic floor, hip rotator, and hip adductor muscles, working your muscles to the point of fatigue. You might feel your muscles quivering during the exercise, or after you're done. If so, you've done it right!

You might also feel an emotional release during or after the series, as the psoas (hip flexor) and inner thigh muscles are regions that tend to house chronic muscular tension and even emotional energy from the past. This series incorporates ideas from The Revolutionary Trauma Release Process by David Berceli, Ph.D.[64]

Berceli has proposed that by activating the body's natural tremor process in these deep pelvic muscles, a resulting "release" will travel through the body wherever chronic tension is held. This is based on the premise that the psoas (hip flexor) muscles originate at T12 and L1-5, a region that's highly concentrated with sympathetic nerve fibers. The sympathetic nervous system is activated especially under conditions of stress, and by evoking trembling (and then relaxation) in this powerful sympathetic center, an outward radiation and release of other parts of the body that hold emotional trauma and/or muscular tension may be evoked. See www.traumaprevention.com for more information about Berceli's technique and research.

FROG SQUATS (REPEAT): After the "Hip Activator Series," rock yourself up (hands behind your thighs and exhale) and move back into the starting position for "Frog Squats." Complete another 10 repetitions.

STANDING HIP CIRCLES: Stand tall, feet hip- or shoulder-width apart, and circle your hips around 10 times to the right, and then 10 times to the left, as if you're drawing a circle on the ground beneath you. Try to keep your head and shoulders still throughout.

This fluid, feminine exercise gets you out of linear, straight-plane movement. It activates all of the hip and core muscles and can prevent back pain if completed regularly.

PELVIC ROLL-UPS: In standing, lift one heel and bend the knee of that leg. Scoop your pelvis by tucking your tailbone under and then rolling up, one vertebra at a time. Pop your bottom back and your bust forward as you reach the top of your "roll-up." Complete 10 roll-ups, then switch sides and repeat.

"Pelvic Roll-Ups" lubricate the spinal joints and energize the core.

REMINDER: View the digital workout online at www.femfusionfitness.com/energizer.

GODDESS PLIÉ SQUATS INTO DEEP GROIN STRETCH: Begin in a wide-leg plié position (knees and toes pointing outward). Zip up your core muscles and lift your arms, as if you're holding a large ball over your head. Don't let your back overly arch; pull your lower ribs in if they pop forward. Complete 5 plié squats, inhaling as you squat down and exhaling as you press up.

After 5 squats, squat down again and sweep your arms down, pressing your forearms into your inner thighs. Press out and back to stretch your inner thigh and groin regions for 15-20 seconds. Rock gently side to side, if you wish.

The "Goddess Plié" strengthens the quadriceps and hip adductors as well as the buttocks and pelvic floor. Holding the arms overhead serves to further activate the deep core muscles, lights up the upper chakras, and makes this a more functional exercise than a squat on its own.

SEXY SQUATS: Turn your feet so they are facing forward and bring your feet shoulder-width apart. This time when you squat down, sit back as if you are sitting into a deep chair. Really stick out your rear! Do not let your knees go beyond your toes. As you sit back, arch your spine and look up toward the ceiling. Let your hands travel down from your thighs to your knees as you inhale and sit back into the squat.

To return to a standing position, tuck your tailbone under, look down toward the floor, and tighten your buttocks as you round your back toward the ceiling. Let your hands travel up your thighs and exhale as you round up to stand.

Complete 5 slow, sexy repetitions.

This exercise should be slow and controlled. Take your time with it, and vamp it up! There's nothing sexier than a woman who knows how to linger.

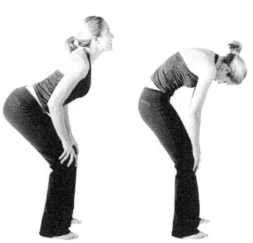

Sexy Squats

PLIÉ SQUAT WITH HIP CIRCLES: Return to a wide-leg plié position (knees and toes pointed outward). Place your hands on your hips or in a "prayer" position in front of your heart. "Re-zip" your core muscles, and circle your hips 10 times to the right and then 10 times to the left. Stay low, in a plié squat, the entire time, as you circle your hips. Be sure your knees do not drift inward. Keep the knees tracking directly over your 3rd and 4th toes.

This isometric squat is solid through the legs, but fluid through the hips and spine. It strikes a beautiful balance between fluidity and control. Imagine the hip circles moving energy up through your entire chakra system, from the first (base) chakra, up through the second (sacral), third (solar plexus), fourth (heart), fifth (throat), sixth (third eye), and seventh (crown) chakras.

SUNSHINE BREATH INTO FORWARD FOLD: Stand with feet hip-width apart and hands at your sides. Inhale as you wing your arms out and up overhead. Exhale as you wing your arms out and down, and then walk your hands down your legs to the point where you feel a stretch in the backs of your legs (your hamstrings). If you have any back pain or history of spinal injuries, place your hands above or below your knees for support. If you do not have pain or history of injury, cross your arms and let your head hang, really stretching and releasing your hamstrings. Breathe deeply and relax into this stretch for 15-20 seconds. To finish, bend your knees slightly and inhale as you wing your arms up overhead, returning to a standing position. Fill your entire being with light, from your fingers to your head and down your body into your toes before returning your hands to your sides. Repeat 2 times.

This is the final exercise in the Inner Core Energizer routine. The purpose is to stretch the spine and the backs of the legs, to balance the energy between the right and left sides of your body, and to feel energy pulsing and moving throughout your chakras.

REMINDER: View the digital workout online at www.femfusionfitness.com/energizer.

Summary of the Inner Core Energizer:

Pelvic Rocks: 30-60 seconds

Pelvic Bounces: 30 seconds

Stirring the Pot: 5 times each direction

Open Like a Book: 3-5 times each direction

30-Second Breath Meditation

Bridge with Block into Deep Abdominal Wake-Up: 3 bridges, followed by 10 wake-ups

Long Leg Stretch: 5 times each side

V-Legs: 10 repetitions

Butterfly Bridge: 10 repetitions

*Prance into Deep Ab Blaster: 10 prances, followed by 10 blasters

Bridge with Hip Circles: 5 circles each direction

Slalom: 20 repetitions

Superwoman with Foot Taps and Mini Rear-Lifts: 3 repetitions of the entire sequence (10 foot taps and 3 rear-lifts)

Child's Pose All Directions: 15-20 seconds in each position

Kneeling Foot/Toe Stretch with Hands Clasped Overhead: 15-20 seconds

Chest Expansion: 15-20 seconds

Kundalini Heart Opener into Bust Circles: 20 heart openers, followed by 5 bust circles each direction

*Naughty Cat into Rocking Horse: 10 naughty cats in each direction, followed by 10 rocking horses on each side

Kneeling Series: 10 hip pumps, 5 hip circles each direction, 5 wide-knee kegel lifts

Side Plank with Oblique Twists: 10 twists each side

*Plank with Hip Drop: 10 hip drops each side

Downward Facing Dog with Alternating Knee Bends: 30 seconds

Pigeon Pose: 30-60 seconds each side

Deep Squat with Kegels: 30-60 seconds

Frog Squats: 10 repetitions

Hip Activator Series: 3 minutes total

Frog Squats: 10 repetitions

Standing Hip Circles: 10 circles each direction

Pelvic Roll-Ups: 10 each side

Goddess Plié Squats Into Deep Groin Stretch: 5 squats followed by 15-20 second stretch

Sexy Squats: 5 slow and sexy squats

Plié Squat with Hip Circles: Hold squat while circling hips 10 times each direction

Sunshine Breath into Forward Fold: 2 repetitions, holding the forward fold for 15-20 seconds each time

*See notes for women with diastasis recti (DR).

Chapter 14

FOOD PHILOSOPHY

"When diet is wrong medicine is of no use.
When diet is correct medicine is of no need."
–Ayurvedic Proverb

The primary goals of this book are for you to understand and appreciate your body and to provide you with a safe fitness routine that will leave you feeling radiant, sexy, and strong. However, *Lady Bits* is ultimately a lifestyle program, and a well-rounded lifestyle program is not complete without addressing food and nutrition.

CLEAN EATING AND BIOINDIVIDUALITY

I am a firm believer that a happy belly leads to a healthy, happy, energetic mind and body. I fully respect that every person's physiology is slightly different and that not everyone responds to the same diet plan for improved health and wellness. There are very few hard and fast rules that work for everyone, but there is one that I feel should be "gospel" for all individuals: **eat food as close to its natural state as possible**. Processed food laden with chemicals, syrups, colorants, and preservatives should be banned from grocery shelves and most certainly from your kitchen cupboard.

I told you a bit about my health journey at the beginning of this book, but I think it's time to tackle another aspect: my food journey. At risk of sounding like a complete basket case, I want to share it with you in order to highlight the importance of feeding your body appropriately (whatever that means for YOU, because remember, everyone is different).

Flash to in image of me curled into a ball, sobbing hysterically on the floor of my toddler son's bedroom. HE had to comfort ME. It still makes me shudder thinking of that moment.

Now flash back even further, to me as a young adult. I'd always had digestive troubles growing up, but it wasn't until I was in my late teens and early twenties that my lifestyle choices and stress began to wreak havoc in my life. I couldn't think clearly, I was forgetful and lethargic, and I sunk into a deep clinical depression that required therapy and medication.

Thanks to my mother's encouragement, I consented to medical testing for gluten intolerance that included gene analysis and a stool sample. The results were clear: I had a raging case of gluten and dairy sensitivity, as well as the genes linked to celiac disease. Finally, I had an answer to why I always felt so sad, mentally foggy, and generally "off:" the food I had been eating my entire life was linked to my mental health issues. I had grown up eating pasta, bagels, and as much cheese and yogurt as I could get my hands on...and now it was time to stop. Once I eliminated gluten and dairy, the sunshine came back into my voice. I gained energy and felt much better, but to be honest...I still wasn't 100 percent.

Time went on. I graduated from demanding college and graduate school programs, got married, and had my son. I looked healthy on the outside, but I still suffered bouts of anxiety and depression. It didn't hit home that I needed to do something MORE about my food and lifestyle choices until that fateful day on my son's bedroom floor. I was wracked with tears and he was comforting ME, saying, "It's okay, mommy," and hugging me...hanging on for dear life. It was a pivotal moment. I realized that if my toddler had to take care of me, there was something seriously wrong that I needed to figure out.

With the help of a naturopathic doctor (and hours upon hours of my own research and experimentation), I uncovered additional foods that I am sensitive to and adopted a much "cleaner" whole foods diet that is now basically grain-free and legume-free, as well as gluten-free and dairy-free. When I keep my food choices in-check – combined with managing my stress, understanding my body and my hormones, and staying active as we have discussed thus far – I feel better today than ever before. Although I still have good days and not-so-good days (the ups and downs of life are unavoidable), my baseline level of health and mental wellness is on a much higher plane. I will never, ever look back to my days of pizza and cheese-smothered noodles.

Now hear me out: I love food! I do not subsist on a boring, bland diet of kale and poached chicken. I read cookbooks from cover to cover, poring over the photos and imagining how I'll tweak the recipes to make them my own. To me, food and cooking is not just about nourishment; rather, it's a form of creative expression, of joy...of art!

To many people, my gluten-free, dairy-free, soy-free, and mostly grain-free diet might seem limited and restrictive, but for me, it's anything but. I've learned how to cook and enjoy delicious "clean" food that makes my body feel and look its radiant best.

"What is clean eating, anyway?"

This is such a great question, since many people – including myself – throw around the terms "eating clean" and "clean foods" frequently but LOOSELY. We don't always provide a solid definition of what eating clean actually looks like.

My first experience with (what I now consider to be) truly "clean" eating was about 15 years ago at Red Mountain Resort and Spa in St. George, Utah. I saved up my money and embarked on a young single gal's **fabulous adventure** that I expected to include massage and luxury and loads of delicious food. Although I got all of those things, I wasn't expecting such simple fare:

- Steamed vegetables that sung without any sauces or "extras" added.
- Bountiful salads with simple oil and vinegar dressings.
- Seared meats, cooked to perfection.
- Sparkling water with a twist of lime.

I will never forget the meals that were so simple, yet so flavorful.

I'll also never forget the cooking class I took at Red Mountain. The chef made a sweet potato chiffon pie that was squeaky clean, gluten-free, grain-free, and dairy-free. Of course, those things didn't mean anything to me at the time...I just knew that it tasted amazing despite the fact that the crust was made primarily of crushed nuts and the silky filling was low in sugar with ingredients that were simple, raw, and natural.

At the time, I was NOT eating that way at all. Cereal, chips, instant noodles, and packaged pancake mix were staples in my college apartment. **Now, 15 years later, I know what clean eating is and I know why it's so incredibly important for our health.**

Clean eating has different meanings for different people based on the diet that works best for them. For people who follow a vegan diet (with no animal products), free-range chicken eggs and raw, unpasteurized honey will not be "clean." If you're Kosher, the most humanely raised pork will never fall into your personal guidelines of clean eating. **But the commonality between all "clean" diets is this: it's REAL FOOD that comes from the earth.** It does not come from a package or a box. It does not originate in a factory. It originates in nature.

I'm a huge believer in bioindividuality. Everyone's nutritional needs and food tolerances vary, but we can all agree that if it's not from nature, proceed with caution. If it has loads of ingredients and/or ingredients you can't pronounce, if it's shelf-stable for years on end, and if it was lab or factory created...don't eat it. It's not good for your skin, your body, your teeth, your brain, or your waistline.

Registered dietician Beth Danowsky, RD, encourages her clients to do most of their shopping on the perimeter of the grocery store (which, in the United States, tends to house produce, meats, seafood, eggs, and dairy). But sometimes you need to venture into the interior, where more packaged and processed items tend to be held. Beth follows three simple rules when purchasing from the interior of the grocery store. Begin by looking at the label. First, the item should contain ten ingredients or less. Second, you must be able to pronounce each ingredient (and know what it is). Third, the first three ingredients should not be sugar in any of its hidden forms, from corn syrup to cane sugar to dextrose, maltose, or fructose. Remember: even "organic sugar" is still sugar!

Here's another way to determine if a food item is "clean:" if you can find it in the coupon section of your weekly newspaper, it's probably not clean. The hard truth is that clean foods are often NOT on sale. But you'll triple your savings if you eat clean by boosting your immunity, feeling "clearer" mentally, assisting your body in healing naturally, and avoiding unnecessary trips to the doctor.

FOOD SENSITIVITIES

I want to take a moment to discuss food sensitivities. Eating anything your body is sensitive to can cause inflammation, mood issues, skin issues, and GI distress. More than 75% of all people have some kind of food sensitivity or intolerance.[65] Discovering if you have any can help cure nagging and long-term health issues and can help you look and FEEL your best.

> **Fun Tidbit:** Did you know that inflammation can cause puffiness and water retention? Many people lose 3-5 pounds within just a week or two when they eliminate a food that their body is sensitive to, even if they change nothing else. It's like magic!

Here are some of the most common food sensitivities:

- Gluten sensitivity is suffered by up to 1 in 7 people, or 15% of all individuals.[65] Gluten is the protein found in wheat, barley, and rye. Estimates of the prevalence of gluten sensitivity range, but it is generally accepted that there is a spectrum of gluten sensitivity from mildly intolerant (which may affect a higher percentage than 15%), to the most devastating form, celiac disease (which affects a much lower percentage). Although there may not be a "perfect" answer when it comes to the prevalence of gluten intolerance, suffice it to say that MANY people are affected by it.

- The inability to fully digest milk products (dairy sensitivity) affects up to 75% of all people.[65] Both lactose (milk sugar) and casein (milk protein) can be troublesome. Thus, if you suspect a dairy sensitivity and don't experience relief when you consume "lactose-free" dairy products, you might actually be sensitive to casein.

- One in three people (approximately 33%) experience sugar sensitivity – most commonly due to fructose malabsorption.[65] Fructose is found in fruits, of course, but it is also found (and is usually super-concentrated) in processed foods like soft drinks and sweets. High fructose corn syrup, and even "natural" alternatives like agave nectar are two of the top offenders. Most sugar sensitivity goes undiagnosed, but it can be responsible for symptoms like stomach bloating, diarrhea, dehydration, unexplained weight loss and other intestinal distress. These are the kind of symptoms that we dismiss in our busy lives by taking over-the-counter medications!

- Up to one in three people (33%) suffer from yeast sensitivity and/ or candida overgrowth, which can manifest as recurring yeast infections, skin problems such as athletes' foot and ringworm, lethargy (extreme tiredness), severe sugar cravings, and GI problems (flatulence, bloating, constipation, or diarrhea).[65] What is candida? Candida albicans are parasitic fungi that resemble yeasts. They are usually benign, but when the conditions are right (or wrong, as it were) they can become pathogenic and grow, unchecked, throughout the mouth, vagina, skin, and intestinal tract. Yeast and fungal overgrowths are often an indication that you have additional food intolerance(s) and that your gut is in distress. If you've experienced yeast and other fungal infections that come back again and again, you need to let go of yeast-containing foods like breads, rolls, and bagels, and then work with a qualified healthcare practitioner to determine if you have any other food sensitivities that are contributing to your condition.

HOW FOOD AFFECTS YOUR MOOD

Did you know that your gut actually produces and transmits neurotransmitters that we used to believe were only produced and contained within the brain? It's true! As much as 95% of your serotonin is contained in your gut.[66] Serotonin is responsible for calmness and pain reduction. **The healthier your gut is, the healthier your response to stress and pain.**

The correlation between the health of your "gut microbiome" and your mental health is fascinating. I'll just share a bit, briefly.

Microbiome literally means "little world," and it's like that in your gut! There are tens of trillions – up to 2 kg or 4.4 pounds – of microorganisms in every person's gut.[67] These tiny little microorganisms are a lot like people; they're all different. There are at least 1000 different species of known bacteria, each with their own genetic identities. As stated in an article on the gut microbiome, "One third of our gut microbiota is common to most people, while two thirds are specific to each one of us. In other words, the microbiota in your intestine is like an individual identity card."[67]

Just like human beings, some of these microorganisms are "good" and others are a tad unsavory. In a healthy gut, the good guys (good bacteria) displace the bad guys (bad bacteria) that can invade your body and cause inflammation and ultimately, disease. You need to eat healthfully to support the good guys! Healthy bacteria protect the fragile cells of the gut lining, they synthesize certain vitamins, and they ferment foods that aren't digestible.

You are as healthy (and happy) as your gut, and supporting your "good" gut bacteria is key. Feed them quality, nutrient-dense foods, sufficient fiber, and prebiotics (raw onion, raw banana, or prebiotic fiber blends). You might consider taking a broad-spectrum probiotic to further colonize your gut with "good guys." Talk to your nutritionist, naturopath, or functional medicine specialist for more information.

Another key is keeping inflammation in-check. Inflammation is a subject we covered in Chapter 9 in relation to back pain, autoimmune issues, and more. Although inflammation is essential as a short-term response to injury or illness, chronic inflammation is a bad seed. It can be especially difficult to deal with when the inflammation moves to your brain. **An inflamed brain is an anxious brain!** One of the best things you can do to prevent chronic systemic inflammation is to eliminate (or at least reduce) foods that tend to be inflammatory, such as refined sugar, processed foods, and – for some people – grains and legumes. Crowd out the "bad" foods with clean, anti-inflammatory foods such as fish, berries, and green vegetables. You can also try eating or supplementing with turmeric, which contains curcumin, a potent anti-inflammatory. Research shows that 1000 mg curcumin daily may actually reduce depression as effectively as fluoxetine (the active ingredient in Prozac®)![68]

The overarching take-home message is to EAT CLEAN. Eat whole, nutrient-dense foods and reduce processed and packaged foods. Processed foods may be considered fuel for your body since they provide calories, and therefore energy, but it's dirty fuel. It's like bad gas that makes your engine knock and ping and ultimately shortens the lifespan of your car.

Toss the packaged crackers and cookies. They might be making you depressed and feeling older and less radiant than you actually are.

A few more important clean-eating tips to keep in mind:

- Stay hydrated. I like to start my day with a big glass of lukewarm or room temperature water, sometimes with a spritz of lemon for flavor. This kickstarts my digestion and rehydrates my brain, eyes, and joints which have been away from water all night long. Morning hydration has become one of the most vital parts of my day, and I recommend it to all of my clients.

- Eat breakfast within the first 30-60 minutes of being awake.

- Don't skip meals. Skipping almost always leads to a feeling of deprivation and over-compensation (by over-eating) at your next meal. Maintain a steady blood sugar balance throughout the day by eating every 3-5 hours.

- When you do eat – even if it's just a snack – enjoy a combination of protein, fiber, and healthy fats for maximum satiation and nutrition. See my "Lusty Lady Smoothie" for an example. Ideally, pair it with a hardboiled egg or a slice of nitrate-free turkey or ham.

- Eat locally and seasonally. Produce that's picked in Mexico before it's ripe and then shipped to Canada will not have as many vitamins and minerals as locally grown winter kale when it's kale season. Eating seasonally may mean shifting your taste buds, but it's worth it for the health benefits.

- Healthy food can taste GREAT. When cleaning up your diet, rather than think of all the foods you're eliminating or that you "can't" have, focus instead on what you "can" have. Crowd out the processed, nutrient-poor foods by having plenty of delicious, nutrient-dense foods available at all times. Always be prepared with plenty of fresh fruits and vegetables, olives, raw nuts and seeds, clean proteins (i.e. free-range eggs, grass-fed beef, and wild-caught fish), gluten-free grains and legumes if tolerated, and 70% cocoa content (or higher) dark chocolate. The darker it is, the healthier it is; and on a practical note, it's easier to limit yourself when the flavor is so strong and rich.

- Like routines? I suggest having a big, hearty salad for lunch every day. Simply wash and dry salad greens at the beginning of the week, wash and slice hardy vegetables such as carrots and bell peppers, and prepare a jar of simple vinaigrette dressing. I like to use ½ cup extra virgin olive oil, ¼ cup balsamic vinegar, 2 tsp Dijon mustard, 1 tsp honey, dried herbs such as rosemary and oregano to taste, and salt and pepper to taste. Seal, shake, and enjoy! Make sure you always have protein options available (leftover rotisserie chicken, hardboiled eggs, or broiled salmon). When lunchtime comes around you'll always be ready with prepped greens, veggies, protein, and dressing. Salads are a great way to use random leftovers (i.e. leftover roasted veggies, leftover toasted nuts) and are even better when you mix sweet and salty, crunchy and soft. Throw in some raisins. Sprinkle on some toasted seaweed. Anything goes!

- Grandma was right: chicken soup is a cure-all. Why? Because of the gelatin in the homemade stock (or "bone broth"). Gelatin is a surprising superfood that I encourage you to eat DAILY. Make your own gelatin dessert using well-sourced gelatin and 100% fruit juice or even coconut water. Collagen is amazing for your skin and joints, and it's soothing for your gut lining. If you're healing from any type of food intolerance or gastrointestinal distress, one of the best things you can eat is bone broth and/or gelatin. Look for a brand of gelatin made from pasture-raised cows, such as Vital Proteins™ available at www.vitalproteins.com. You can make homemade broth by simmering the bones and skin from a roasted chicken, for example, and then use the broth in soups or when making braised veggies, sauces, or even as a cooking liquid for rice or quinoa. It's nourishing and anti-aging!

- Speaking of anti-aging, green tea may add years to your life. It's full of antioxidants and polyphenols and has a whole host of other health benefits, including boosting your metabolism. Brew a pot in the morning and drink it throughout the day (green tea does contain caffeine, so caffeine-sensitive individuals may not wish to drink it after 2pm). You can even try giving yourself a facial massage with brewed and cooled green tea for topical antioxidants.

- The single common denominator among all of the competing, sometimes even conflicting, dietary info out there is that vegetables are GREAT. They're naturally gluten free, dairy free, refined sugar free, free of the "bad fats" like trans fats, low in calories, high in fiber, and high in vitamins and minerals. So if you don't already love veggies, learn to.

- Interested in my favorite cookbooks? See the Resources section at the end of the book.

COMMON QUESTIONS

Before we leave the subject of clean eating, I'd like to take a moment to answer some questions I hear regularly.

"Do I need to detox?"

"Detox" is a popular word these days. Did you know that your body is a natural detox-machine? You don't need a 10-day juice fast to cleanse and refresh your system. Every day, particularly overnight, your body "cleans house" and does its best to flush out anything unhealthy or toxic.

It's simple to support your body's natural detoxification pathways, which include the skin, lungs, liver, lymphatic system, kidneys, and intestines. Breathe deeply. Get plenty of sleep. Be sure you're having daily bowel movements. Move as often as possible (walking and twisting motions are particularly good for detoxification). Drink plenty of fresh, clean water. All of the information in *Lady Bits* that you've read – and are going to read – will help.

If you feel the need to get back on track with your health and nutrition goals, or reset your health after a period of over-indulgence, I recommend following a short, food-based cleanse that's based on organic whole foods and plenty of fluids. I recommend my very own *Weekend Reboot* 2-day detox as a safe, effective, and simple solution. See the Resources section at the end of this book for details.

"Are carbs BAD?"

There are no hard and fast rules for everyone. In general (and especially for women), carbs are NOT "bad." In fact, going too low-carb can be hard on a woman's body: it can put your thyroid health at risk, it can shut down your reproductive system (causing you to stop ovulating and plummeting your sex drive), and it can make it harder for you to sleep at night and maintain steady energy throughout the day.

Does this mean that you should go out and stuff white bread into your mouth? No. Stick to the high quality, nutrient-dense, fiber-filled carbs such as veggies, fruit, and starches such as sweet potatoes and potatoes. For those of you who like numbers, low to moderate carbohydrate levels (around 100 grams of carbs per day) are recommended for most modern women who are interested in losing or maintaining their weight. One hundred grams of carbohydrate equates to about four servings of fruit or starchy vegetables per day. For more information, Stefani Ruper offers a great explanation in her book, *Sexy By Nature*.[69]

"Doesn't eating fat make you fat?"

No! Here's a great rule of thumb: lose the sugar, keep the fat.

Sugar is inflammatory, addictive, and completely void of nutrients. Unfortunately, the low-fat fad of the 1980s and '90s persists today, especially amongst women, many of whom still erroneously believe that eating fat will make them fat. Often, low-fat substitutes use sugar to replace the fat in order to enhance flavor. This may be one of the leading causes of obesity, inflammation, and chronic disease that we're seeing today.

Of course, eating too much of any one thing isn't ideal, but eating fat in and of itself does not make you fat. In fact, fat is necessary for proper absorption of certain vitamins and minerals. Fat is what your brain cells are made of, so it will improve your mental clarity and efficiency. It keeps you feeling calm, grounded, and satiated. It's a slower burning energy source. Furthermore, as discussed in Chapter 9, fat is required for proper production of sex and stress hormones.

In a nutshell, fat is fantastic as long as you choose high quality fats such as extra virgin olive oil, grass-fed butter or ghee, coconut oil, and avocado. Savor and enjoy every single luscious bite. It's not a "guilty pleasure," it's simply PLEASURE!

"I count calories... Why can't I lose weight?"

Weight loss is much more complex than the old adage of "calories in, calories out." Rather than counting calories, the best thing to focus on is the nutrient density of your food choices. When you choose low-calorie foods that are devoid of the micro- and macronutrients your body needs, your body will hang on to excess weight and experience cravings night and day. Thus, you'll hang on to stubborn weight!

If you must count something, count nutrients. Again, Stefani Ruper offers further details in *Sexy By Nature*.[69]

"I read a book that said I should (insert nutrition advice here). Will that help me?"

There is as much nutrition advice as there are stars in the sky. When determining the best course of action for you, I encourage you to really step back and take a look at your life (from a practical standpoint), you personal preferences, and your history of strong needs and desires when it comes to food. From there, you can decide which pieces of nutrition advice to take and which to leave behind.

Eating a clean, whole foods diet is not a short-term solution. There is no end-point or end-goal in mind. Rather, eating clean is a lifestyle choice, so you need to make it your own in order to make it work. **Don't force yourself to fit in the mold of someone else's plan.**

Eat clean in a way that works for YOU. For example, I have heard – within a clean-eating framework that otherwise works well for me – that starting your day with a green smoothie is a nutrient-dense, time saving approach to breakfast. But I know that for me, this is not sustainable or realistic. I need solid food for breakfast; I wake up hungry, and a smoothie alone just doesn't cut it unless I'm doing a focused (short-term) food-based cleanse such as my *Weekend Reboot*. On a daily basis, I feel best when I start my day with a hearty, whole-foods breakfast that is higher in carbs than what I eat later in the day. It's just the way my body works. I still listen to – and learn from – others, and I'm open to experimenting with new information and ideas, but I do so within a framework that is realistic for me.

Rather than following someone else's "rules," I encourage you to do what feels good for you.

Let that sink in... Do what feels GOOD.

Are you worried that if you really and truly took that advice you'd end up gaining 500 pounds because you'd be stuffing yourself with cookies and never moving a muscle? I beg to differ. If you're honest with yourself... really honest about what feels good in your body and what makes you feel your best physically, emotionally, and spiritually... you will naturally – and intuitively – treat yourself right.

One reason you might be stuck feeling not-so-good today is that you consistently reach for food items, plans, and programs that you think will make you feel good, but they end up making you feel terrible. On one end of the spectrum this could be short-term blasts of gustatory happiness, such as the second or third helping of dessert. On the other end of the spectrum this could be starving yourself, or overly restricting yourself, because you think it's the "answer."

Really consider, "Will this make me feel GOOD?" Whether it's a restriction or an indulgence, this question will center yourself and return you to your personal needs and intuition. When you receive an answer, trust yourself and follow your instincts. Sure, there might be a "breaking in" period when you overeat junk and lie on the couch all day, but little by little, as you continue to commit to doing what feels good, the junk will fall away and it its place will be (internal) wisdom and clarity – that is individualized and different for every person – to help you reach your highest potential.

This is your life; don't feel like you have to fit into someone else's box. Pick and choose what works for YOU, and create a personal dietary approach that best suits your needs. You might need to start with a done-for-you plan and then branch off as you get to know your body and understand the concepts of eating in a clean, unprocessed, nutrient-dense way. But making it your own and listening to your instincts is truly the key when it comes to making sustainable change.

My friend and mentor Jessica Drummond coaches her clients to: "Eat the best [highest quality and most nutrient-dense] food you have access to with complete pleasure and enjoyment. **Stressing while eating even really healthy food may reduce its goodness!** Pleasure is KEY."

Just like exercise, if you're not enjoying your healthy diet, you're never going to stick with it. Healthy living isn't about deprivation; rather, it's about learning how to enjoy the process of making better choices for your body. I promise – once you see how RADIANT and ALIVE clean eating makes you feel, you'll never want to go back.

Find a healthy eating plan that makes **your** body feel great, and then stick to it...for life. Your body does a lot for you; do your part to treat it (and feed it) well.

HEALTHY FOOD IS SEXY

This is a shining example of clean, plant-powered, whole foods goodness. Read about the health (and libido) enhancing benefits of each ingredient as you savor every sweet-tart sip and the subtle notes of rich cocoa.

Lusty Lady Smoothie Recipe
(serves one)

Add to blender in this order:

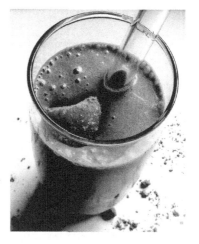

- 1 cup almond milk

- 2 Tbsp unsweetened 100% pomegranate juice

- Heaping ½ cup frozen raspberries or strawberries

- 1 Tbsp extra virgin coconut oil

- 1 Tbsp unsweetened cocoa powder

- Optional: 1 tsp organic raw honey or 5-8 drops liquid stevia

When you start to blend, use a low speed. It takes time to move the larger chunks of fruit to the blades. Gradually increase speed to high as this happens.

Blend on high for 30-45 seconds, or until completely smooth. Add a splash of additional almond milk if needed, to allow for easy blending. Serve immediately.

Did you know you have an apothecary in your kitchen? These are the health (and libido) enhancing benefits of the Lusty Lady Smoothie:

Almonds are high in antioxidants, calcium, and magnesium. They are have a low glycemic load, which helps prevent blood sugar spikes.[70] The almonds in this recipe are consumed in the form of almond milk. Use store-bought almond milk or homemade. Homemade is ideal, as it contains only two ingredients: almonds and water. Simply blend 1 cup almonds with 4 cups water for 2 minutes on high, and then strain through a fine mesh "nut milk" bag. That being said, store-bought almond milk is a convenient option and one that I often resort to, myself. I always have a carton of packaged almond milk on-hand for those times when I run out of homemade and just don't have the time, energy, or ingredients to make more. **Always remember, it's not about being "perfect," it's about doing the best you can, being easy on yourself, and enjoying yourself along the way.**

Historically, **pomegranate** has been a symbol of fertility. It has now been shown to decrease hot flashes and possibly even increase sperm motility (so if you're hoping to conceive, have your husband drink this smoothie, too).[71] The nitric acid in pomegranate helps blood vessels relax, making it great for heart health and for promoting healthy blood flow throughout the body, including the erogenous zones. Furthermore, pomegranate antioxidant levels are through the roof and in animal studies, pomegranate extract has been shown to slow the absorption of sugar into the blood.[70]

Raspberries are anti-inflammatory and contain a compound called ellagic acid, which may inhibit development of certain cancers. They are high in resveratrol (also abundant in red wine and cocoa powder) which may inhibit certain neurological diseases such as Alzheimer's and Parkinson's, and might even help to slow the aging process by delaying normal cell death.[70]

Strawberries are rich in vitamin C, which aids in the production of collagen, which is vital for skin health as well as smooth, wrinkle-free skin. Like raspberries, compounds in strawberries have been shown to kill certain cancer cells and help normal cells repair themselves.[70] **When purchasing strawberries, be sure to purchase organic. Strawberries are known to be highly absorbent of pesticides. They are consistently one of the top offenders on the "dirty dozen" list (published every year by the Environmental Working Group).**

Coconut oil is known to be anti-inflammatory, and get this – it's also an antiseptic! Coconut oil is an outstanding source of lauric acid, which has antibacterial, antiviral, and antifungal properties.[70] **Did you note that this recipe calls for an entire tablespoon of coconut oil?** This is not a misprint. Many nutrition experts encourage women to eat MORE fat (healthy fats, such as coconut oil), using a guideline of approximately 1 Tbsp per meal of health-promoting fats such as coconut oil, avocado, olive oil, grass-fed butter, and/or ghee.

Cocoa powder (and cacao, which is the raw, less processed form of cocoa) contains flavonols that may prevent coronary artery disease, reduce blood pressure, reduce insulin resistance, and protect red blood cells.[70] Dark chocolate is also an excellent mood enhancer... **Enjoy, lusty ladies.**

Chapter 15

MINIMIZING TOXIC LOAD

I am not trying to scare you, but it's not just what you ingest – what you surround yourself with also affects your body and your health. There's no need to run for the hills to start living in chemical-free caves, but it's important to be informed and aware.

We are exposed to alarming amounts of toxins in our environment every single day, from the air we breathe to the water we drink...not to mention the products we slather on our body and spray around our home! Human bodies are required to handle and process more toxins than ever before and our organs of detoxification can only take so much. In addition to feeding ourselves the nutrients we need in order to add health and vibrancy to our lives, we also need to REMOVE some of the toxic substances that – cumulatively – are doing us (possibly a lot of) harm.

Plastics are one of the worst offenders and as time goes on, plastics are found in more and more forms, in more and more places. Bisphenol A (BPA), a component of many plastics used for food and drink storage, has been discovered to be an endocrine (hormone) disruptor. In recent years, plastics companies have jumped on the opportunity to create BPA alternatives so that they could label their plastics "BPA-free." Unfortunately, BPA alternatives such as Bisphenol S (BPS) may disrupt normal brain cell growth, and have also been tied to hyperactivity in children, even in extremely low doses.[72]

Strangely, even seemingly innocuous things like receipts can contain BPA and BPS. Some scientists are now warning everyone, but especially pregnant women, to steer clear of plastics, including handling receipts, due to the endocrine-disrupting effects and effects on neurodevelopment.[73]

I'm not an expert in toxin-free living, but in my opinion, any step you take to reduce your toxic load is a step in the right direction. Here are some of my priorities:

- I store my foods in glass storage containers rather than plastic. In addition to glass containers I've purchased, I save and re-use glass jars (i.e. spaghetti sauce jars, jam jars, coconut oil jars) for storing foods such as leftover olives, sliced carrots, and coconut milk.

- When on-the-go, I always use glass water bottles. I love Lifefactory® bottles (www.lifefactory.com), since they're encased in rubber to prevent breakage.

- I load up on cilantro. Cilantro is a known heavy metal chelator (it binds toxic heavy metals such as cadmium and lead and removes them from your body), and has been proven in mouse studies to protect the kidneys and bones from exposure to toxins.[74] I add cilantro to salads, guacamole, homemade salsa, curries, and soups. Try making cilantro pesto: Simply replace half (or all) of the fresh basil with fresh cilantro in your favorite pesto recipe.

- I take my food sensitivities seriously in order to protect my intestinal lining. A strong intestinal lining prevents entry of toxins into the body via "leaky" junctions in the gut, which can occur when food sensitivities remain unchecked.

- For household cleaning, I use a homemade all-purpose surface cleaner with a 2:1 ratio of distilled white vinegar and water in a spray bottle. This ratio is sufficient to cleanse and kill germs without harming your health. I usually add a few drops of lemon and rosemary essential oils, and use this blend to clean my kitchen and bathroom counters and other non-porous surfaces.

- For their natural beauty and their powerful air-cleaning abilities, I bring houseplants into my living environment. Some of the best choices for natural air purification include: English ivy, spider plant, peace lily, Chinese evergreen, bamboo palm or reed palm, snake plant, various varieties of philodendron and dracaena, Gerbera daisy, chrysanthemum, and rubber plants.[75]

- I make every effort to purchase personal care products such as soap, shampoo, and conditioners that are gluten free, paraben free, and phthalate free.

- Here's a fun trick – to kill odor-causing bacteria, I prime my armpits with a swipe of rubbing alcohol and witch hazel, then apply nontoxic deodorant (I enjoy Primal products, from www.primalpitpaste.com).

- Clean and simple is my motto. The fewer ingredients, the better. I use pure, organic coconut oil to cleanse my skin and remove mascara, and pure, organic jojoba oil to moisturize my skin after my shower.

- I say "no thank you" to receipts, when an option is presented.

For loads of free information about low-toxin living, I encourage you to check out the blog www.wellnessmama.com. At the time of this writing, there are entire sections dedicated to "Natural Home," "Beauty," and "Remedies" that can help reduce the toxic load for you and your family.

Chapter 16

THE 80/20 RULE

You have to be willing to invest time and effort into your health, and true, it takes some planning and extra work. However, you don't have to be "perfect" to be healthy.

The *Lady Bits* way of living is not just about living healthfully, it's also about living happily. While not yet recognized in the DSM-V (a manual used in the medical fields to classify psychiatric diagnoses), orthorexia nervosa is a type of eating disorder that is becoming more and more prevalent. As written by Karin Kratina, PhD, RD, LD/N on the National Eating Disorders Association (NEDA) website:*

"Orthorexia starts out as an innocent attempt to eat more healthfully, but orthorexics become fixated on food quality and purity. They become consumed with what and how much to eat, and how to deal with 'slip-ups.' An ironclad will is needed to maintain this rigid eating style. Every day is a chance to eat right, be 'good,' rise above others in dietary prowess, and self-punish if temptation wins (usually through stricter eating, fasts and exercise). Self-esteem becomes wrapped up in the purity of orthorexics' diet and they sometimes feel superior to others, especially in regard to food intake. Eventually food choices become so restrictive, in both variety and calories, that health suffers – an ironic twist for a person so completely dedicated to healthy eating. Eventually, the obsession with healthy eating can crowd out other activities and interests, impair relationships, and become physically dangerous."[76]

*Please note that the NEDA does not consider orthorexia nervosa an official diagnosis, nor are they pushing to have it included in the next edition of the DSM. More information about NEDA is available at www.nationaleatingdisorders.org, and their toll-free helpline can be reached at (800) 931-2237.

The 80/20 Rule is an excellent way to live a healthy life that doesn't shift into the realm of orthorexia. It's all about balance. The idea – when applied to healthy living – is that if you make the best possible choices 80% of the time, you can enjoy some flexibility 20% of the time...and do so happily, without a trace of guilt.

Although 100% commitment to healthy living might be your ultimate intention, you cannot – let me repeat, cannot – be "strict" or perfectly compliant 100% of the time. Let's face it...life happens! This is not an easy excuse; it's simply a reality check.

Furthermore, the value of making a "bad" choice every once in a while – whether due to unavoidable circumstances (such as being stuck in an airport with limited food options) or due, pure and simply, to a desire to indulge – is that it shows you how far you've come, and usually, how much you don't want to go back to where you were before!

My husband was finally able to stick to a healthy eating plan when he allowed himself one day per week of indulgence – eating anything he wanted without shame or guilt. When he first started doing this, he went a little crazy on his "free" days. Every time, he felt so bloated and ill after his day of debauchery that he was reminded of why he had chosen to eat healthfully in the first place.

Today, my husband and I live in a delicious state of balance. We eat a clean, whole foods diet Monday through Friday, with zero refined sugar and limiting (or eliminating) alcohol. On the weekends, we loosen up and allow potato chips (my personal weakness) or French fries into our lives, a couple of glasses of wine, or some other indulgence. It's not perfect, but it's healthy (overall) and sustainable for the long haul.

The 80/20 Rule offers a forgiving and realistic approach to healthy living. The key is personal commitment to living the *Lady Bits* way. Give it 100% and know that it's okay when you make a poor choice, enjoy a treat, or when "life happens." When you shoot for 100% and end up at 80%, you'll still be well on your way to sustainable success and a lifetime of health.

A FemFusion friend stated:

"80% of the time I don't eat anything processed. 20% I either haven't found a good replacement or I'm just am not willing to give it up yet. I will say that the ratio has slowly changed. When I started [eating clean], I think it was the other way around, but slowly I've found more and more ways to eat real food more often."

I encouraged her to stay right where she is. Going too far beyond 80/20 can feel cloying and restrictive. Who wants that?

Chapter 17

MINDSET

We've talked about setting a baseline of health by getting plenty of rest and relaxation, moving more, eating clean, and minimizing toxic load, but do you know the most important element for creating a foundation of health? It's your mindset. Believing that life – in general – is good and worth living, believing in your own value and your God-given right to health and happiness, and trusting that the universe is out there to support you.

> **"Once you make a decision, the universe conspires to make it happen."**
> **–Ralph Waldo Emerson**

Mr. Emerson may have been one of the first promoters of "The Secret!" Whether you believe in the Law of Attraction or if you think it's just a bunch of New Age hype, you've got to admit...what you think about repeatedly usually happens. Keep your thoughts as positive as possible.

A positive mindset is crucial for living a sustainable healthy lifestyle. You must have faith that if something bad is happening – if there's a bump in the road such as illness or injury, or a setback that causes the proverbial sh*t to hit the fan – there's a lesson or a gift to learn from.

> **"We need to accept that we won't always make the right decisions, that we'll screw up royally sometimes – understanding that failure is not the opposite of success, it's part of success."**
> **–Arianna Huffington**

As happiness expert Marci Shimoff states, "Don't believe everything you think." She reports that the average person has 60,0000 thoughts per day, and 80% of them are negative.[77] We inherited this "negativity bias" from our caveman ancestors; in order to survive, they needed to be aware of the fears, the dangers – essentially, the negative – in their lives. But today, even with our full bellies and our comfortable homes that are (usually) free from the threat of lions or tigers lurking nearby, this negativity persists, and often unnecessarily. Because of our built-in "negativity bias," our minds tend to grab on to negative thoughts, whereas positive thoughts slide right off.

Test yourself – if you get 10 compliments in a day and 1 criticism, what do you remember? If you're like most people, you focus on the critical remark. Happier people reverse that tendency.

> **Fun Tidbit:** It takes MUCH LONGER to register a positive thought than a negative, so you really have to stop and RECEIVE the positive. When something good happens, or when you get a compliment, savor it. Let it land. Digest it. Take it into the cells of your body. Spend a solid 30 seconds accepting, allowing, and cultivating this positivity.

Begin to focus more of your attention on the positives and less on the negatives. This attention creates new neural pathways in the brain that will allow you – the next time things take a turn for the worse – to return more quickly and easily to the positive aspects of life.

Gratitude practices help with this. Take a few minutes every day to think of – or better yet, to write down – three to five things you're thankful for. Everything from the great breakfast you ate to the cashier who smiled at you. Setting aside time for gratitude causes you to STOP long enough to take it in and actually register the good.

> **"The subtle secret to possessing all you want:**
> **blessing all you have."**
> **–Mike Dooley**

Another fun exercise is to copy the phrase "Something wonderful is about to happen!" on sticky notes, and place these notes throughout the house. You might be surprised to find that they catch you off-guard and fill you with the same anticipation and excitement that a child feels on Christmas Eve: "What's the surprise? What's it going to be?"

"Yeah right… I wouldn't fall for a sticky note."

If you're a skeptic or if you feel negativity set in, chase it away with a simple, "Well… What if it's true?" Because you never know: this could be the day that something miraculous truly DOES happen.

Clear your mind, be open to possibility, focus on the good, and expect positive things to come into your life. This mental, emotional, and most importantly – energetic – shift is essential for your health and happiness.

> **"If you have good thoughts they will shine out of your face like sunbeams and you will always look lovely."**
> **–Roald Dahl**

PERMISSION TO ADJUST YOUR SAILS

Two important things to keep in mind; first, what works for you one day might not work the next. Second, a soul-satisfying, healthy lifestyle will look different from one woman to the next.

It all comes down to listening to your intuition. Check in with your mind, body, and soul on a regular basis and be willing to adjust your lifestyle choices relative to your individual needs. This is something to take seriously, especially as women with our delicate hormone balance that CHANGES over time, and even from day to day with our monthly cycles.

As important as exercise is, any type of physical exercise is a stress to the body. Remember that there are "good stresses" and "bad stresses." Exercise is definitely a good stress, but it's still a stimulus that creates a physiological response. Your heart rate goes up, certain stress hormones are released (especially in more intensive activities), and your body's ability to cope with these physiological stressors can change based on time of the month, other stressors in your life, and age-related changes.

"I've heard of women who run marathons in their eighties. How come they can run long and hard into old age, but for me, running feels like torture?"

Just because an exercise program works for someone else does NOT mean it's (necessarily) going to work for you. Likewise, just because it worked for you five years ago doesn't (necessarily) mean it's going to work for you today.

On a similar note, you might thrive on an extremely low-carb diet in your twenties or thirties. But over time, you might discover that this way of eating no longer serves you. You might feel fatigued and less vibrant than usual. If so, no matter how "healthy" your lifestyle appears on paper, it may no longer be the healthiest choice for you at your current age and/or stage of life. You might need to add some healthful carbs back into your diet, such as sweet potatoes or gluten-free grains.

The take-home message is that if you really LISTEN to your body, you will hear it speaking to you. Take the time to watch for cues and to honor your needs. You can always experiment with something new and go back to your old ways if it doesn't work out, but know that it's normal and natural for your needs to shift and change over time. Roll with it!

> **"We turn not older with years, but newer every day."**
> **–Emily Dickinson**

PART V:
Love Your Body

**WE COULD ALL USE
A LITTLE MORE PLEASURE
AND A LITTLE LESS
SELF-DEPRECATION
IN OUR LIVES.**

"Beauty begins the moment you decide to be yourself."
–Coco Chanel

*"It is just as time consuming and difficult to learn to accept yourself as it is
to pretend to be someone else. The only difference is – with self acceptance,
one day, it's not hard anymore. One day, you feel like your sexiest,
strongest self just rolling out of bed in the morning."*
–Vironika Tugaleva

"Love yourself first and everything else falls into line."
–Lucille Ball

Chapter 18

LOVE YOURSELF FIRST

What's ten times more important than eating your greens, taking probiotics, or getting to the gym? What's far more essential than sitting in meditation, getting enough sleep, or doing your kegels?

Self-love.

It's foundational to a healthy, thriving, radiant life.

I'm going to say it again: self-love. What does the term "self-love" bring up for you? What feelings or images does it invoke? Does self-love seem self-indulgent, entitled, selfish, or hedonistic? Is self-love scary, nebulous, woo-woo – or more likely – is it something for other people, but not for you?

You might think that physical intimacy with a lover is the ultimate act of vulnerability, but I beg to differ. Sure, a partner can reject you. But have you ever rejected yourself? Worse, do you reject yourself all the time?

"God, I hate my body."

"I'll never look as good as her."

"She's so much better at (fill-in-the-blank) than me, anyway."

"It doesn't feel safe to stand out."

"I can't change... I just can't. Besides, what will they (do, think, say) if I really start to be the woman I know I really am?"

Before you can open yourself sexually, mind, body and spirit...before you can look someone in the eye and really own what you have to say...before you can accurately see what the mirror reflects back to you...before you can feel embodied as a woman and see the magic that truly is all around you...you must love yourself. **Heck, before I could write the words on this page and really mean them, with my whole heart, I had to love myself.** I know this journey because I've lived it. I'm still picking my way through the cobblestones today.

Only with self-love will you value yourself enough to stick to a lifestyle program that supports your health, will you forgive yourself when you screw up, and will you see your value reflected in the eyes of another.

We are all so very, very different on the outside, but I believe that deep down, at the core of our beings, most women have similar desires: a desire to feel beautiful and wanted, and a need for passion in our relationships and our lives. How often have you coveted another woman's shining hair? How many tubes of "miracle cream" have you purchased to smooth your cellulite or create porcelain skin? How many times have you wished that your lovemaking could be as passionate as it appears on the silver screen, or that your life – in general – was as fulfilling as it seems to be for your friends?

> **Before you can clean the house, you have to see the dirt.**
> **The brave first step is knowing that there could be MORE,**
> **and being willing to explore it.**

Sometimes we're so busy chasing all the things we haven't got that we forget to recognize the beauty that is already within and around us. **Be grateful for what you already have. This creates space for even MORE radiance to come into your life.** Love, understand, and accept your body (and your life) FIRST; the tight abs and great sex come second.

THE UPSIDE OF SENSITIVE

I identify as a highly sensitive individual. I am hurt easily, I internalize, and I am very, very hard on myself. I overthink almost everything, and I have an energy level that is highly vibrational. Due to the plethora of connections in the traditional feminine brain, this is a common trend among women.

In the past, I considered this highly sensitive nature to be one of my greatest weaknesses but now I consider it to be my greatest strength. Not only do I have a deep inner life that is fascinating and unique, I am also able to identify with other women. I am able to appreciate and value all the unique sides of myself. I'm fiery, I'm passionate, and I'm unpredictable... I'm a beautiful, radiant woman regardless of what I look like on the outside.

Through investigating my own sensitive, intricate nature I have uncovered my insecurities and have actively worked to dismantle them. As I discover more and more about who I am, chipping away at my old emotional blocks, I become more "me." Feminine. Powerful. Grounded in my identity.

Check in with yourself: Have you done the (inner) work?

Before you can fully open yourself to your partner, before you can be present with them in all your radiant glory, you must surrender to the vulnerability of opening up to YOURSELF; of really looking at yourself, and loving and accepting yourself no matter what you see. This deep inner work will awaken the radiant, sensual goddess within.

LEARNING HOW TO "BE"

"All of humanity's problems stem from man's inability to sit quietly in a room alone."
–Blaise Pascal

Do you ever just sit and "be?" I'll admit, this is hard for me. A favorite quote of mine is, "The quieter you become, the more you can hear," (Ram Dass). But this takes practice and a certain level of comfort with stillness and being alone with yourself.

When I began a dedicated practice of being with myself, within 30 seconds of sitting I'd start to feel prickly and crawly, and my mind would wander to everything else I needed to do. I'd feel tension in my chest and my head would start to pulse. My mind was willing to be everywhere but there...with everyone else, but myself...on every task but the quiet task at-hand.

> **"The truth is, anyone who's meditated even one day, learned fast, that we almost are never present."**
> –**Pema Chödrön**, in *Heart Beats: Music-Infused Insights*[78]

Over time I developed the ability to sit and just "be" for 5-10 minutes at a stretch, which did wonders for my mood, stress level, and my ability to be gentle and accepting. It's almost as if during these moments of "Brianne time" I developed a strong friendship with myself...one of those deliciously comfortable friendships where you don't always need to speak, yet the silence is never awkward.

Just like any relationship, you'll want to take this slow. You wouldn't proclaim love or "best friend" status to an acquaintance; rather, you would take time to get to know him or her first. Sure, you've "known" yourself your whole life, but how often do you take the time to focus on YOU? Do you really know who you are? Are you comfortable with your thoughts and your personality? Sitting in silence can feel strange. "Stuff" can come up...stuff that can make you want to stand up and distract yourself with something external. Before we move on to more in-depth self-love practices, we need to learn how to simply sit and BE.

I mentioned "stuff" coming up. We've all felt it...moods, anxieties, fears, anger, sadness, and the never-ending to-do list. I like to equate "stuff" to clouds in the sky. If you have ever been a passenger in an airplane you'll know that above the clouds, there is always clear blue sky. If you live in cloudy climates you might think of sunny, blue sky days as transient: a condition that comes and goes like the rest of the weather. But the reality is that blue sky is constant. It's the other "stuff" that passes through – the clouds, the rain, the snow, the hail, and the turbulence you feel as your plane descends. What's above the ever-changing weather patterns? Without fail, above the clouds is pure, brilliant, clear blue sky.

When learning how to be with yourself, the aim is to see beyond the clouds (the "stuff" of daily life) and recall the beautiful blue sky that is always within.

"I close my eyes in order to see." –Paul Gauguin

Let's begin with an exercise that will help you learn to embrace stillness, and ultimately, learn how to be comfortable being still, quiet, and alone with yourself...even if only for five minutes. A few minutes of stillness is so simple, yet it's a profoundly therapeutic tool that anyone can access, anytime of the day, and use it to release old patterns, center yourself, and connect with yourself.

EXERCISE – Sitting and "Being:"

The following are three visualization meditations that I like to use; choose the variation that works best for you. The body position is the same for all, but the hand position is different. For all variations, you will sit in a comfortable cross-legged position with your back straight. This will be easier to do once your core muscles gain strength by way of the Inner Core Energizer routine (Chapter 13). If it's uncomfortable for you to sit cross-legged, you can sit in a straight-backed chair that has armrests. I suggest setting a timer for five minutes, so you won't worry about the time or about falling asleep.

<u>If you tend to be more lethargic and fatigued, or if you lack motivation, then try this variation:</u>

Sit as described, with your hands on your knees if cross-legged, or resting on the armrests if in a chair. <u>Turn your palms up (see photo)</u>. This is an energizing mudra (hand position) that represents <u>receiving energy and inspiration</u>. Begin breathing slowly and deeply. Allow your inhale to expand the back and the sides of your ribcage, and down into your abdomen and pelvic floor. As you exhale, *gently lift your pelvic floor and pull your lower belly inward. This is Core Breathing, as described in Chapter 11. Focus on this breathing pattern, taking it slowly and gently. As you breathe, imagine ascending toward the heavens. Your thoughts are just clouds passing by, as your consciousness travels up, up, up, above the clouds, into the clear blue sky. Maintain the visualization of the cloudless sky for five minutes.*

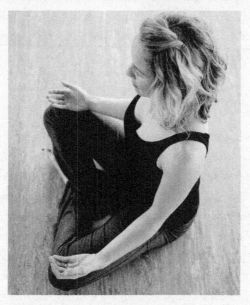

Hand position if you tend to be lethargic and fatigued

If you tend to be more high-energy, anxious, and "head in the clouds," then try this variation:

Sit as described above with your hands on your knees (if cross-legged) or resting on the armrests if in a chair. <u>Turn your palms down (see photo)</u>. This is a "rooting" or "grounding" mudra that can help <u>still and calm</u> the mind. Begin breathing slowly and deeply. Allow your inhale to expand the back and the sides of your ribcage, and down into your abdomen and pelvic floor. As you exhale, gently lift your pelvic floor and pull your *lower belly inward. Focus on this breathing pattern, taking it slowly and gently. As you breathe, imagine a deep blue ocean. Your thoughts are the waves on the surface of the ocean. Sometimes these waves are just ripples, and sometimes they're 30 feet high...but the ocean is vastly deeper than even the tallest waves. Allow your consciousness to travel down, down, down, past the waves, into the depths of the seemingly infinite clear blue ocean. Maintain the visualization of the calm, deep sea for five minutes.*

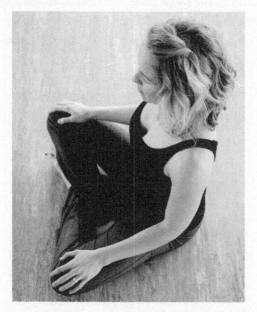

Hand position if you tend to be anxious and high-energy

If you're not comfortable with water, then try this variation (also done with your palms facing down):

As you breathe, imagine a bustling city on the surface of the earth. Picture yourself as a large oak tree outside the fast-paced city. As you begin Core Breathing, visualize your massive, ancient trunk and your strong, burrowing roots growing down, down, down into the warm, rich, brown soil.

The center of the earth is thousands of miles away. Grow down – root down – as far as you can, and then stay there. Maintain this visualization for five minutes.

Fun Tidbit: Snatch small moments. Does the word "meditation" conjure images of saffron-robed monks sitting in silence for hours on end? Meditation doesn't have any requirements or trappings such as candles, incense, chanting, or 45-minute segments of time. Rather, you can catch small moments throughout your day to try the exercises above. The next time you park your car, take a few minutes to be still and just "be" before getting out and moving on with your day.

"To find peace on top of a mountain is easy, to find peace in the chaos of ordinary life is true enlightenment."
–Laura Bell Bundy

Chapter 19

BODY IMAGE BOOTCAMP

Now that you're moving toward a place of being comfortable, quiet, and still with yourself, let's get to the heart of the matter: your body image.

Imagine what it would be like to be completely free from anxiety about your body and your appearance. To accept yourself just as you are. Wouldn't that be amazing? Wouldn't it feel free?

Improving your relationship with your body helps you feel free in your love relationships, as well. Your relationship with YOU will improve your relationship with everything – and everyone – around you. Unfortunately, many women imagine themselves to be inadequate or deficient in at least one – if not several – areas of their lives, usually including their appearance.

There are thoughts that serve you and thoughts that don't. As spiritual leader Eckhart Tolle teaches, you have a (thinking) mind, but you are NOT your mind. Not everything you think is true, and not all of your thoughts (in some cases, very few of your thoughts) are helpful and productive when it comes to your health and well-being.

Polly, one of my health coaching clients, opened her heart to me stating:

"I have a deplorable self image. I can remember hating my thighs in first grade. It has been made even worse by the weight gain and body changes from pregnancy and birth. I love my daughters — I think they're better than perfect — and I want them to see themselves like I see them. What can I do to teach them that being beautiful and healthy is inside of them, not in their jeans size? **[I know that] confidence and loving yourself is just as important as everything else, and that's where I have so many issues.** *How do I convey loving who you are? I don't want them ever worrying about their weight or the size of their thighs."*

Polly nailed it. If you don't love yourself, you won't respect yourself enough to treat your body properly with nutritious food and regular exercise. What's more, you won't be the best possible role model to your children.

It shows when women don't love themselves. They don't sparkle with confidence. Rather, they shrink and fade, dimming their own light because they don't want others to see the "horrors" (real or imaginary) that they see in themselves.

But here's the thing: the true path to radiant beauty is not looking like a supermodel. The key to radiant beauty (and sex appeal) is self-confidence, **and this comes from self-love**. When you love yourself – even the shadow parts of yourself (on a mental/spiritual level) and the parts that you or society have deemed "ugly" or imperfect (on a physical/external level) – you'll naturally make healthier choices and better decisions when it comes to your health and well-being. This will transform your external appearance and will cause you to shine from the inside out.

The best part? Others around you will notice, and most likely, will want to follow your lead. The super-duper best part, especially for mothers of daughters? You will leave a legacy for them, a legacy that will serve them – and their children – well into the future.

LIGHT AND LOVE MEDITATION

Meditation has been proven to effectively decrease anxiety while increasing creativity, focus, and compassion. The following **five minute light and love meditation for body image and negative self-talk will not only help you, but others around you will be affected by your positive energy and inner radiance**.

> "When one is out of touch with oneself,
> one cannot touch others."
> –Anne Morrow Lindbergh

EXERCISE – Light and Love Meditation:

Begin with Core Breathing (Chapter 11). Find the spot in your body that is holding the most tension, insecurity, self-judgment, or even self-hatred. Is it somewhere on your face? Is it in your chest? Is it your belly or your thighs? Is it your hips or your pelvic area? Is it your sexual organs? Focus on these tension-filled areas and observe any negativity or judgments as they come. These judgments and negative self-talk might be about appearance, or they might be about function (or perceived lack of function).

As you observe the judgments and negative self-talk, visualize filling the area with a warm golden light and think the word "love." Spend one to two minutes letting the sensations of light and love grow and expand.

As this sensation and visualization of light and love grows and expands, bring the focus back to your breath. Breathe out the judgments and tension, and breathe in even more light and love.

When you feel relaxed and warm, move on to the next area of your body that holds tension and/or insecurity and repeat the meditation.

I love examples, especially when things are a bit nebulous and intangible (like all visualization and meditation techniques initially seem, in my opinion). If you do not understand the Light and Love Meditation, read through the following example.

Light and Love Meditation Example:

Jen lies down on her couch and begins Core Breathing. She mentally scans her body and notes the first thing that comes to mind. The first thing Jen notices is a feeling of tightness and constriction in her chest. It feels like a band that is preventing her from breathing easily. She focuses on her chest. She observes her thoughts; she had a rough day at work and starts thinking of the stack of papers that remain in her inbox. She allows this observation. She allows her anxiety, and the judgment that comes along with it ("This is crazy; I need to let it go. Why can't I just relax? I'm so damn uptight!"). She does NOT try to dismiss or ignore her thoughts and fears; rather, she envisions a warm ball of white light that starts small in her chest and slowly grows as she continues Core Breathing. She begins to slowly repeat – like a mantra – the word **love**. The white light and the feeling, vibration, and sense of the word **love** expand, and soon her chest and shoulders are enveloped in warmth and good feelings. As the light and love continue to expand, she breathes out the dark judgments and tension with every exhale. With every inhale, she breathes in even more love and light. This continues for one to two minutes. When Jen feels free of tension in her chest, she moves on.

Jen feels relaxed, warm, and vital in her chest and the feeling of constriction has disappeared. She continues to mentally scan her body. Her mind "stops" on her thighs. **She hates her thighs** – she is terribly insecure about them. She thinks her cellulite is like a neon sign that her husband can't help but notice when she is nude. She allows these thoughts, but also asks that they come gently so as not to overwhelm her. She continues Core Breathing as she focuses on her thighs. She allows her insecurities and the judgment that comes along with her thoughts ("If only I could lose five pounds... Why can't I stick to my diet? What's wrong with me?"). She does not try to dismiss her thoughts; rather, she envisions a warm ball of white light that starts small in her pelvis and slowly moves down her thighs as she continues Core Breathing. She begins to slowly repeat – like a mantra – the word **love**. The white light and the feeling, vibration, and sense of the word **love** expand, and soon her entire pelvis and both thighs are enveloped in warmth and good feelings. As the light and love continue to expand, she breathes out the dark judgments, tension, and insecurity with every exhale. With every inhale, she breathes in even more love and light. This continues for one to two minutes. When Jen feels free of anxiety and judgment about her thighs, she moves on.

As Jen continues to scan her body, she notices that she feels wonderful. She is relaxed and warm, and feels positive and secure. She slowly opens her eyes, rests for a few more seconds, and then moves on with her day.

NOTE: This meditation is particularly effective for pain. If you have areas of pain, such as your low back, your hips, or your sexual center (i.e. dyspareunia or pain with intercourse), sending love and light energy to these regions is one of the most healing things you can do. Any time you focus your awareness on a part of the body, it increases circulation. This can work wonders when it comes to relaxation and release of tight, tense muscles.

GET REAL... GET NAKED (MIRROR WORK)

Getting to know yourself is not an easy task, and it's one that scares many women to the point that they won't take a step forward. They get stuck here, and may not even be able to identify that their health journey is deadlocked in self-avoidance! But often, a lack of self-love and a lack of self-acceptance is the very thing that's holding them back from reaching their full potential of radiance. Stubborn weight, lingering ailments, and unconscious resistance to making healthy changes (which often leads to self-sabotaging behaviors) can all stem from low self-worth and poor body image.

When it comes to loving ourselves just as we are, many of us disown, reject, and push ourselves away. We forget the freedom we felt when we were children and loved our bodies as-is. We loved running around, buck naked, without a care in the world. Although clothing is great, wouldn't you like to reclaim that sense of freedom and complete "okay-ness" with your body and the world around you?

Daily visualization and meditation practices (such as the preceding examples) are a great start, and journaling – simply free-writing whatever comes to mind – is another fantastic way to get to know your true thoughts, feelings, and needs.

But I want to get a little more concrete. **To really love your body, you**

need to see yourself.

Check in with yourself: What do you see when you look in the mirror? What comes to mind? Are you able to hold your own gaze?

A mirror is just a piece of glass. It simply provides a reflection of your image that your visual cortex – and then the rest of your brain – interprets. Any judgment about the image comes entirely from you, possibly including, and certainly not limited to: Expectations, past hurts, regrets, and old stories.

So again…what do you see? Do you see your mom's nose – the nose that she always hated? Do you zoom in on your eyes that your Aunt Glenda said were too closely set?

I've already shared the "negativity bias" that is hardwired into so many of us. But just as shifting to a positive mindset is essential for health and happiness, a positive – or at the very least, a neutral (as a starting point) – mindset about yourself and your body is essential for establishing a baseline of self-love.

> **It's not your body that causes you pain,**
> **it's your THOUGHTS about your body.**

The next time you look in the mirror, try looking at yourself as an outsider would, without judgment, criticism, or old stories. Focus on coming from a neutral perspective. Then hone in on one thing that you love. Maybe it's your eyes that have garnered a few compliments over the years…or your hands that are so capable…or your strong, square shoulders…or the single dimple that shows when you smile.

The following mirror exercise is based on the work of Louise Hay, a beacon of light in the world of personal development.[79] Hay's classic book, *You Can Heal Your Life*, inspired this exercise, which is about seeing who you really are when you're not caught up in rejecting yourself.

EXERCISE – Mirror Work:

The first step is to look at yourself in the mirror, fully clothed, fully made up (if you typically wear makeup). Look into your eyes and say "I love you" and then insert your name.

"I love you, (your name)."

Remember to breathe. It's amazing how often we hold our breath when doing something confronting or uncomfortable!

Notice what you're experiencing. Study your reflection...and your reaction.

Do you laugh nervously? Do you feel ridiculous? Do your eyes betray feelings that you didn't even know you had? Do your eyes say, "Yes, I really do love you!" or do they question the statement? If so, try again. Say, "I love you (name)." You can say it out loud or in your head, whatever is more comfortable (although out loud is more powerful). Think about why you love yourself by stating one thing about yourself that is unique and fabulous and perhaps different – or more outstanding – than other people you know.

Now try, "I love you, (your name). You are ADORABLE." Or, "I love you, (your name). You are such a powerful woman." Or perhaps, "I love you, (your name). You are so strong, and a fantastic mother." Or maybe, "I love you, (your name). You are healing me, and I am so grateful."

When saying "I love you" with makeup becomes easy, strip off a layer. Look at yourself without makeup and say, "I love you (name)."

When this becomes easy – granted, this could take weeks, don't be hard on yourself – remove an item of clothing and

To take this exercise even further, and to make it even more powerful, incorporate touch. Gently touch and explore your body, especially in places you don't like, or places you'd rather avoid. Touch the cellulite on your thighs. Touch your genitals. Touch your stomach. Touch your stretch marks.

Looking at – and touching – your body can bring up shame and vulnerability, even with yourself…even when you're completely alone. But through vulnerability comes TRUTH, acceptance, and freedom.

Remember Polly, the woman who focused on her thighs and was concerned about passing her negative body images to her children?

Here's her follow-up after working on various exercises related to self-love and self-acceptance:

"I can't tell you what a significant moment it was to discover – at 36 years old – that I had FINALLY started loving myself. I cried. (I ugly cried.)

Since that moment I've really tried to focus on myself in a positive way and I can't believe the difference… I now see my body as something miraculous and I think it's responding. I'm not even doing anything physical right now, but I know that the response is attributed to my new state of mind. My body and my mind are finally becoming friends and I've never felt that before. I want to be better and healthier because of it. I feel more womanly, fiercer, stronger, definitely more connected to myself… It's like I finally figured out how to turn on my superwoman switch.

And I get to have incredible moments, like last night. My 19-month old is teething again and having problems sleeping. She's big for her age, so standing up and holding her for hours isn't an option anymore. I took her into the playroom and laid with her on a big, plush beanbag. She snuggled up against me, draped over me, with most of her body on my stomach and chest. And she just stared at me with a sleepy gaze. Every time I switched positions with her, all she wanted to do was snuggle up against my stomach. It's the place she likes to be. Even though it's getting smaller, my stomach is still soft and mushy... It's like her personal pillow. I finally love that. Before, I would have been self-conscious. I would have focused on the wrong thing and would have missed out on a very beautiful moment between my baby and me. I've learned that it isn't enough to be physically healthy; you have to be 'love-healthy,' too. And I'm on my way."

MEET YOUR INNER CRITIC

The mirror exercise might have brought up some issues for you. If so, great! You have to uncover your deep-seated issues in order to dismantle them.

Making healthy changes that last can be challenging, and you've GOT to have support. You need good people on your team...and the captain of this team needs to be YOU. Self-sabotage via negative self-talk can hold you back from realizing your dreams and shining to your fullest potential.

It's time to meet your inner critic – your inner "mean girl," as I like to call her. Shine light on your inner mean girl and then try something new. Stop yourself when you think or say something critical in order to reprogram and "clean up" your old, self-limiting beliefs. Your inner mean girl is another name for FEAR, and rather than stuff it, it's better to bring it into your conscious mind. If you don't, she (i.e. your fear) will unconsciously drive your behaviors and actions. She will encourage you to eat the entire pizza, or look at your body with harshness and anger, or stay in bed all day rather than join your family for a hike. **It's always better to be driven by love than to be driven by fear.**

EXERCISE – Meet Your Inner Mean Girl:

<u>Step One:</u> *Personify the negative voice inside your head – the*

voice that is preventing you from reaching your goals (or has held you back in the past). Give her a face. Give her a name. One of my clients visualized a sassy little girl with a mop of bright red hair who stood with her hands on her hips as she spouted negativity. Another client saw a lizard-like creature with hard, mean eyes and a forked tongue. My inner mean girl looks a lot like me, except that her eyes are harsh and critical, always judging. She often comes up when I'm doing the mirror work described above, trying something new, or preparing to launch something big (like this book).

Step Two: Don't try to fight your inner critic (your inner mean girl). Negativity is STRONG, and often wins. Instead, befriend her. Let her know that you're a strong woman, too. Offer to take her to tea, or out to lunch, or simply to sit in the sun and have a friendly chat. Discuss your dreams and ask if she can help you reach your goals. Often, bullies are lonely and just want attention. They may be fearful of your burgeoning strength and power. Give her some attention...show her some love...and more often than not, she'll leave you alone.

If that doesn't work, then get mad. Get crazy. Let loose, and let her have it. As a previous client stated:

"I met my mean girl on the scale. I had been trying to embrace her and love her, but instead, I removed her and her throne completely out of my bathroom and replaced it with a full-length mirror directly across from the tub! The number on the scale will NEVER define who I am again."

One of the major lessons I have learned is that it can be scary to grow into your own power...to lean into your own light, and to release the shadows within that can hold you back from reaching your full potential. You might need help feeling the truth that it's safe to feel confident and strong.

Two techniques that can help are prayer and the Emotional Freedom

Technique (EFT), commonly referred to as "tapping." EFT is far beyond the scope of this book, but I am living proof that it works. See the Resources section at the end of the book for more information about EFT/tapping.

The following (non-denominational) prayers were inspired by skincare expert Fran Kerr of www.highonclearskin.com.[80] The first is directed at self-love, and the second specifically relates to releasing your inner critic. Recite either prayer while looking at yourself in the mirror. Do this three times per day for the next 30 days and expect a major shift in self-perception.

Option One: "I release and let go of these patterns of a lack of self-love and a lack of self-confidence. By Divine Grace, these patterns are released here and now. Thank you, thank you, thank you; it is already done."

Option Two: "I release and let go of the inner critic who inhabits my body and my mind. She does not serve me, and she never will. By Divine Grace, she is released here and now. Thank you, thank you, thank you; she is already gone."

TURN IT OFF TO TURN IT ON

As Dr. Joy Jacobs – a clinical psychologist and expert in body image and eating disorders – relates, our culture is surrounded by images of the "skinny body" ideal. Although in recent years there have been campaigns to stop the practice of airbrushing, and to feature plus-sized models, there is still minimal acceptance for diversity among body types in mainstream media. That's why, in early stages of treatment, Jacobs counsels her clients:

"Do not read magazines. Cancel your subscriptions, turn off the TV, and start paying attention to the variety of body types even among your closest friends and family. Think of the people that you love most and that you feel best around. Does it have to do with them looking a certain way or being a certain size? Ninety-nine percent of the time it has nothing to do with any of that."[26]

Rather than focus on looks and physicality, Jacobs asks her clients, "What do you want to be remembered for?" She continues, "Do you really want to be remembered as the one who wore the size zero jeans, or do you want to be remembered for who you are, how you lived your life, how you loved others, how you loved yourself, and what that did to serve others?" [26]

Your body is not what gives you love in this world. Answer these questions for yourself right now. What is your body here to do? What are you here to be? How do you want to be known? When you have the answers, place them in your heart, and then throw out those lingerie circulars and celebrity tell-all magazines. Turn off the television. Screen the images you'll allow "in."

Turn it off, and then turn it on.

EXERCISE – Find Beauty Everywhere:

Start to notice the good in other people's bodies... "Regular" people's bodies. Notice the beauty in the curves and the intrigue in the imperfections. Often, it's easier to see the beauty in others than it is to see in yourself.

This exercise is powerful and can be done anytime, anywhere. On the subway, at the grocery store, or even in certain forms of media (for example, magazines dedicated to plus-sized or older women). But as you notice other women around you, beware of two "old friends" that can creep in: judgment and jealousy.

Rather than comparing and judging in a harsh way (which is actually the act of bringing others down in order to bring yourself up), or envying others who seem to have, be, or look your "ideal," try to open your mind and see only beauty. I promise, when you really look with an open mind, open eyes, and an open heart, it will make you want to cry tears of joy at the radiance of it all.

"And I said to my body, softly,
'I want to be your friend.'
It took a long breath and replied,
'I have been waiting my whole life for this.' "
–Nayyirah Waheed

Chapter 20

OWN YOUR FEMINITY

As a woman, you are magnificent in your own rite. Your curves and feminine features are naturally sacred, sensual, and beautiful. You are not an object that needs to look a "certain way," and it's ABSOLUTELY what's on the inside that counts. Everything in the previous section on self-love and self-acceptance reflects that message. But owning your femininity is easier – and more satisfying – when you take some pride in the outside, too.

I have found that to really open up my "goddess channel" – to feel my most radiant, my most sexy, and my most confident – I must take at least a modicum of care in tending to my personal appearance. This really hit home the day I skulked into my son's piano lesson to pick him up, wearing a dirty sweatshirt, three days worn yoga pants, not a stitch of makeup, and hadn't showered in over 24 hours. My son's put-together piano teacher did a double take, looking at me with a mixture of pity and embarrassment that she tried her best to hide...but I saw the sad reality of how I was treating myself reflected in her eyes. It was then that I realized that I'm in my mid-thirties, and it's no longer "cute" to lounge around in my pajama pants all day long like I did as a college co-ed (but then again, was it ever cute?).

This isn't to imply that you must only go out of the house if you're fully made-up and coiffed. **For me, however, it means that I make it my personal mission to get out of my workout clothes after my daily exercise session.** Since I work from home, this task is surprisingly easy to skip! I usually only "step it up" to jeans, or "nicer" yoga pants, but at least they're clean. It also means that at the very minimum, I'll put on a swipe of mascara and a dab of my favorite essential oil blend. Why? Because it makes me feel my best.

Check in with yourself: What do you need to do, appearance-wise, to feel your best? Whatever it is, are you doing it on a regular basis?

THE RED NAIL POLISH CHALLENGE

Last January, my New Year's Resolution was to wear (unchipped) red nail polish every day for the entire month. Although it was a bit of a hassle to keep my nails looking their best, this simple act of self-care and honoring my femininity was the best thing I did for myself that month. Even when I was wearing my sweat pants, I still felt like a vixen.

Whether it's red nail polish or a lacy bra, challenge yourself to step up your game in a small way – maybe even a secret, for-your-eyes-only way – that makes you feel feminine and sexy. The spillover effect from these small actions can be astonishing. Give it a try and see for yourself!

Walk down the street with your head held high. Look people in the eye when you enter a room. Own it. Work it! You deserve it.

MOVE LIKE A LADY

A huge component of my FemFusion® Fitness classes includes shakin' it in a room full of women with only two rules:

- No judging yourself or others.
- Have fun.

We move our bodies in fluid, circular, sometimes humorous – but always feminine – motions including hip circles, booty pops, bust slides, and shimmies. I act as a guide, showing participants the general technique for these feminine movements, but from there, it's about FEELING the rhythm of the music and the movement and learning how to trust your body…learning how to feel and sense every beautiful muscle and joint, learning how they move and work together, and trusting yourself to move fluidly and sensually without a second thought about what others might be thinking about your body or how you look. I refer to this as "moving like a lady." Men can certainly shimmy and circle their hips, but it looks (and feels) a lot more natural for women to move their bodies in this way. I encourage my participants to "own it" and it never fails that they walk out of their FemFusion class feeling sexy and feminine even though they're dripping with sweat.

If you don't have access to a FemFusion class in your area, it's just as fun to do this at home. Alone. In your undies (or even less). Release your insecurities, move like a lady, and feel free, sensuous, and beautiful.

Put on your favorite music – whatever makes your hips start moving and your body start flowing to the rhythm. From Bach to the Beach Boys to Bruno Mars, it doesn't matter – just move your body to the beat. **Don't worry about how you look, just focus on how you feel.** This exercise can be incredibly freeing if you're willing to take it to the utmost level and do it nude. Grab a space heater if your room is chilly, blast those tunes, and lose yourself in the music. Unleash the wild, creative, dance-hungry goddess inside. There's nothing more liberating or loving you can do for your body or yourself.

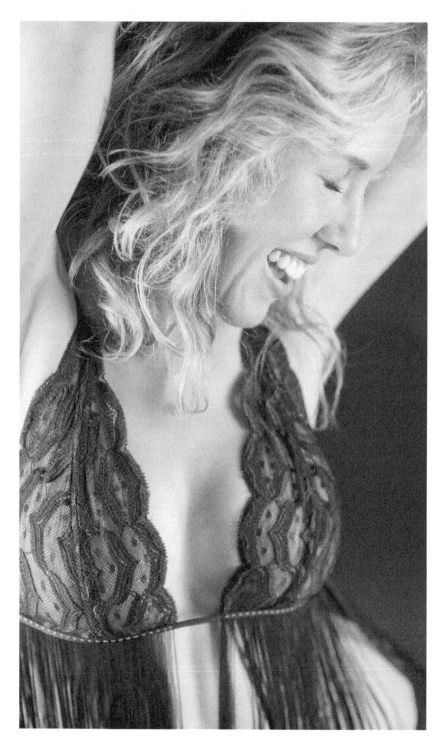

Lady Bits

Self-love: Yep, it's hard (for many women). And no, it's not common.

It takes deep inner work – which could be as simple as the exercises described above, or as complex as years of therapy – to learn how to really love and appreciate yourself for who you are on the inside...not just what you look like on the outside. Sadly, 80% of women in the United States are dissatisfied with their appearance.[81] **But, as I hope I have made clear, in order to truly be sexy inside and out – to really embody your radiant, sexy self and to unleash your inner goddess – you need to love yourself first.** It's foundational to living the passionate, vibrant life you so desperately want to live.

PART VI:
Love Your Love Life

**FEELING GOOD IN YOUR
BODY – KNOWING HOW TO BE IN
YOUR OWN SKIN – IS THE ULTIMATE
PLEASURE-ENHANCING DRUG.
BOTTLE IT UP.**

*"Intimacy – 'into me I see.' Wow, that really woke me up!
Could I find love by looking into myself?"*
–Lisa Nichols

*"Many find it strange for a person to spend their life studying human
happiness and intimacy. I find it strange for anyone not to."*
–Earon Davis

*"It's not true that I had nothing on.
I had the radio on."*
–Marilyn Monroe

Chapter 21

THE *LADY BITS* THREE-STEP SYSTEM

In Parts II and III of *Lady Bits*, you got acquainted with the anatomy and physiology (and even some of the magical secrets) of your beautiful, female body. In Part IV, you learned how to take care of yourself through fitness, proper nutrition, and a positive mental attitude. In Part V, you chipped away at old emotional blocks and learned how to love yourself first; arguably the most important section of the whole program, because if you don't love and value yourself, you won't follow through with any of the positive changes you want to make.

If you have been with me so far, you've created a solid foundation.

Now, in Part VI, it's time to put this knowledge into action and APPLY it toward loving your love life. This section integrates bits and pieces from everything that has led up to this point. Let's get into it.

THREE STEPS TO BETTER SEX

It breaks my heart that so many women struggle with their love lives when so often the answer – and the power to change – lies within. Every woman is a sexual being and therefore suffers on a deep level when she feels she is not the lover she is meant to be. Addressing any issues you have with sex is another important step to being wholly, wildly, beautifully feminine.

I like a system – a plan with a definite course of action, including steps to follow and goals to check off along the way. *Lady Bits* uses a simple **three-step system** that will help you gain body confidence, increase your core strength, and improve your sex life.

- **Step One** focuses on relaxation of the mind and body.
- **Step Two** focuses on targeted core fitness, utilizing the Inner

Core Energizer to fuse strength with sensuality.

- **Step Three** brings it all together and puts the program into practice. You will learn how to use the relaxation techniques from Step One and the strength and coordination gained in Step Two to take your intimate life to the next level.

These three steps are incorporated into the 14-Day Action Guide found in Chapter 24.

Although the work ahead is simple, it will take some time and energy on your part. In order to successfully complete the three steps in the *Lady Bits* program, you must make a commitment to reading the instructions, practicing the techniques, and eventually incorporating each step into your daily life.

A PRELIMINARY NOTE ABOUT PAIN

I discovered that a significant number of women who read my first book, FemFusion Fitness for Intimacy, were drawn to it because they suffered from chronic pelvic pain that often manifested in dyspareunia, or pain with intercourse. These women found the relaxation information in my book to be incredibly helpful – and healing. **If you are dealing with dyspareunia, please focus your attention on Step One (relaxation). Avoid moving on to Step Two (targeted core fitness) until you have been evaluated and treated by a licensed women's health physical therapist or other qualified healthcare practitioner.**

STEP ONE: RELAXATION

The *Lady Bits* three-step program is a systematic approach to help you achieve optimal inner core fitness and wellness of the mind, body, and spirit. This holistic approach to feminine health will enhance your pleasure during sex, your feelings of pleasure and desire, and – most importantly – your confidence. Step One involves relaxation. **Relaxation may feel like a waste of time and a step to skip, but it is one of the most productive and essential things you can do.**

First, before you can feel strong desire and sensations that make you want to initiate (and proceed with) sex, you need know how to relax both body and mind so you can focus your attention on **pleasure**. It is difficult – if not impossible – to feel pleasure when you are focused on the stresses of everyday life. The relaxation training ahead will help you **let go** and be **in the moment**, clearing the mind of excess clutter so that you can focus on the positive!

Secondly, on a physiological level, you need to be able to relax the muscles of your body so that you can effectively and efficiently contract them. Global inner core strengthening and isolated pelvic floor muscle contractions (kegels) will be addressed throughout Steps Two and Three of this program, so knowing how to access and **relax** the inner core is imperative.

> ### Note from clinical experience:
> I once worked with a woman who was athletically built with powerful muscles from a job that required heavy, repetitive lifting. She came to me with complaints of incontinence and lackluster sex. When I checked her pelvic floor muscle strength I was surprised by the results. Her pelvic floor muscles appeared to be incredibly weak; she was unable to do a kegel, and she was unable to feel her pelvic floor muscles when I asked her to engage them. Despite multiple attempts using simple biofeedback and visualization techniques, she still had no idea what I was talking about when I asked her to find and "feel" her pelvic floor. Finally, I realized that this woman could not sense or contract her pelvic floor muscles not because they were weak, **but because they were so tense and tight!** As we completed our initial visit she opened up about a rocky romantic relationship and a huge amount of anxiety related to work. This woman was stressed to the max, and (as is fairly common) she held her tension in her pelvic floor.
>
> We began a program that included manual stretching of her pelvic floor muscles, deep breathing, and various relaxation techniques to allow her mind to slow down and her senses to return to her body rather than the nebulous world of anxiety and stress to which her mind was usually attuned. Slowly, she began to sense

her pelvic floor muscles. We were able to gradually introduce kegels and start training the muscles to increase strength and coordination. Thankfully, her incontinence and sexual issues were largely resolved by the end of our time together.

Relaxation of the inner core muscles can be difficult. For many of us, tensing our inner core is an automatic reaction – it is simply the way we carry ourselves through the day. Have you ever stopped and realized that your buttocks are clenched? If so, your pelvic floor is probably clenched as well. Have you ever felt the need to "suck in" your tummy in order to appear slimmer? Have you ever noticed that you have been holding your breath for (what seems like) hours? If you answered yes to any of these questions, you are not alone. For many people tension is a part of life; something that's carried in their bodies all day long. It can be an unconscious response to the stresses of daily life. Some people hold their tension in their shoulders, some carry tension in their faces...others hold it in their inner core (especially the pelvic floor). Personally, I have carried tension in all three regions – at the same time!

It is normal for muscular tension to increase in response to stress. What is not normal is to retain that tension when the stress dissipates. For some of us, the stress never dissipates. For others, it does dissipate, but our body maintains the tense postures and muscular holding patterns. Even slight sustained contractions can significantly decrease blood flow to a muscle. This is called ischemia, the restriction of blood supply to a body organ or tissue. **Habitually carrying excess tension should not be taken lightly.** It causes muscle pain and fatigue, and ultimately, can cause significant damage and dysfunction to your musculoskeletal system. Thus, ladies, we need to learn how to **relax**.

SENSUAL VISUALIZATION

One of the most delicious ways to relax – with purpose – is with **Sensual Visualization**. The purpose of Sensual Visualization is to use the mind-body connection to increase feelings of sexuality, intimacy, and arousal. Sensual Visualization allows you to take a "time out" from life to think about your sex life and your sensual self, and to really **feel** these thoughts with all five senses. The aim is to whet your sexual appetite.

Let's face it; with our busy schedules, many of us have to plan our romantic escapades. We can be so consumed with family, hobbies, errands, and work that we simply do not take the time to think sweet thoughts... Then when bedtime comes around we are suddenly expected to be "in the mood?" I think not! Sensual Visualization helps you prepare throughout the day by snagging small moments of time to focus on the positive aspects of your partner and your sex life. Replace any negative emotion or anxiety with positive thoughts – memories of your last positive sexual experience, visions of where you were or what you did in the hours before or after.

This can be difficult! Recently, when completing this exercise myself, all of I could think about was my to-do list, the latest "issue" with my son (who is a teenager trapped in a seven-year-old's body), and what I wanted for lunch. But as my own meditation teachers have said, do not be upset with yourself when this happens. Just note the thoughts, gently dismiss them, and continue with the practice.

Take a moment to read through the instructions, and then try it on your own. Sensual Visualization is a lovely way to fuse relaxation and concentration into a titillating, private experience for you to enjoy now (and later).

EXERCISE – Sensual Visualization:

Initiate Core Breathing (Chapter 11) and allow your mind to clear.

Slowly and gently, without struggle or difficulty, recall a positive intimate experience. It does not need to be sexual (although it can be), it simply needs to bring you pleasure when you think about it. Perhaps it was falling asleep in your partner's arms, cuddling on the sofa with steaming cups of coffee in the morning, or an amazing lovemaking experience from your last vacation. As you breathe, focus on that

thought. Recall the surroundings, the feelings, the colors, the
sounds, and the smells. Make it a sensual (as in using all five
senses) experience. If nothing comes to mind, do not feel bad
or alarmed; just relax and let it go. Something will come to
you the next time you try.

After 30-60 seconds of Core Breathing with Sensual
Visualization, bring your mind back to the present moment
and move on with your day.

[Mom, don't read this:] When I practice Sensual Visualization, I always return to the same mind-blowing experience. My husband and I were in a sleeper car of a train, alone on one of our first vacations without our son. It was late afternoon and the warm, golden sun was streaming into our compartment. It was private and snug, and it was hot...too hot for clothes. The car was rocking from riding the rails. It was a strange and heady combination of gentle and yet so, so strong. The sensations were off the charts. I'll leave the rest to your (or rather, to my) imagination.

Please do not feel "dirty" while you are doing this, or worry that you are doing something promiscuous, pornographic, or wrong. All you are doing is recalling memories – it's simple! But what this exercise can do for you and for your relationship is colossal. Some of us have negative associations with sex; we are too tired or we just don't "want it" like we used to, and often we feel ashamed about this. In some cases, sex is painful...and who wants to do something that doesn't feel good? **Sensual Visualization – when completed regularly – can begin to replace negative sexual associations with positive thoughts.** It can help you see your partner in his or her best light. It can bring you pleasure throughout your day...and there is nothing wrong with that!

Again, the "sensual" part of this exercise refers not only to sexuality and desire, but also to "using your five senses" as you think about a positive, intimate, loving memory. It is something you can do at any time throughout your day.

Goal 1: Combine Breath Breaks with Sensual Visualization

- Initiate Core Breathing and visualize a positive intimate experience. Make the memory more vivid by recalling the sensations that were involved in this encounter (sight, smell, touch, sound, and taste).

- Continue breathing and visualizing for at least 60 seconds, then bring your mind back to the present moment and move on with your day.

- Take Breath Breaks with Sensual Visualization every one to two hours throughout the day.

I realize that it can be difficult to remember to take Breath Breaks and to practice Sensual Visualization on a regular basis. However, once these techniques become habits you will start taking breaks without consciously thinking about it. One strategy to remember your breaks (besides use of an alarm or phone application) is to purchase a pack of small dot stickers and place them in various locations that you look at or notice on a regular basis. For example, stick a dot on your bathroom mirror to remind you about your Breath Break when you first wake up, another on your rearview mirror for your drive to work, another on your computer screen to remind you when you get to your office, and another on your refrigerator to remind you when you are in the kitchen.

Taking the time to incorporate these moments of quiet and focused relaxation will work wonders for you both internally and externally. When you relax, your face softens. The worry lines on your face disappear, making your face appear smoother and more youthful. And that glow about you? It's just the Sensual Visualization... Let people wonder.

MOVEMENT FOR RELAXATION

Once you have integrated relaxation into your life by regularly practicing Core Breathing and Sensual Visualization you can further enhance the mind-body connection through a gentle, daily movement routine intended solely for **relaxation**. The following exercises are gentle stretches and movements that relax the inner core and increase blood flow to the pelvic region, both essential components of sexual vitality. Moreover, these exercises improve your personal body awareness, allowing you to physically sense the muscles of the inner core. Developing personal body awareness is hugely important when it comes to increasing self confidence and body confidence, which – in turn – contribute to **better sex every time**.

Complete these exercises every day as you begin Step One of the *Lady Bits* program (relaxation). You do not need to continue with these exercises once you reach Step Two of the program (fitness); however, you may choose to complete them indefinitely if you wish.

The Movement for Relaxation routine includes the following gentle exercises: Pelvic Drop, Pelvic Rocks, and Frog Stretch.

PELVIC DROP (NOT PICTURED): A "pelvic drop" is basically the opposite of a kegel. Remember, it is just as important to know how to relax and release the pelvic floor muscles as it is to know how to contract them. Women who are pregnant need to know how to "let go" in order to give birth. You need to be able to "let go" in order to have pain free intercourse. You need to "let go" to fully empty your bladder. You need to "let go" in order to have a bowel movement! So you see? The release is very important. Give it a try.

Pelvic Drop Practice:

- Imagine your pelvic floor as an elevator that starts at a lobby and can go up two floors, or can go down to a light-filled, completely non-threatening basement. Your baseline level of pelvic floor tension (i.e. no contraction and no relaxation) is the "lobby." Start here. Imagine the elevator doors sliding closed as you begin your pelvic floor muscle contraction. Gently lift your pelvic floor elevator up to the first floor by contracting your pelvic floor muscles halfway. Do not fully contract; in other words, do not allow your pelvic floor elevator to go all the way up to the second floor. Next, relax fully and visualize your pelvic floor elevator lowering past the lobby and going all the way down to the basement. Really, fully, and deeply let go. Release any tension that might be held in the pelvic floor as you imagine the elevator doors sliding open to reveal a light-filled basement. Relax your pelvic floor enough that you stop just short of urinating.

- One of the women in my fitness classes said that the pelvic drop felt so good, "my eyes rolled back in my head!" She was feeling complete and utter pelvic floor relaxation.

- Repeat 5 to 10 times.

NOTE: If you feel like you might actually urinate while practicing this exercise, empty your bladder before completing it so that you feel more comfortable and more able to fully relax the pelvic floor muscles.

PELVIC ROCKS: This gentle, rocking exercise improves blood flow to the pelvic region and is a great way to combine deep breathing with pelvic floor muscle activation. Pelvic Rocks are included in the Inner Core Energizer, but I will describe them in more detail below.

Pelvic Rock Practice:

- Lie on your back with your hips and knees bent. Place your hands on your low belly with fingers touching in the shape of a triangle.

- Exhale and gently pull your abdominal muscles in as you rock your pelvis into posterior pelvic tilt. Your low back will press into the ground and your pubic bones will point up toward the ceiling. The tip of the triangle your fingers have formed will be higher than the base (see picture).

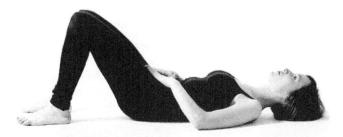

- Now inhale deeply, letting your belly expand, and rock your pelvis forward into anterior pelvic tilt. Your low back will arch slightly and your pubic bones will point down toward the floor. The base of the triangle will now be higher than the tip of the triangle (see picture). As you inhale, notice the gentle downward pressure on your pelvic floor as the pressure in your belly increases.

Allow your pelvic floor to feel the pressure. Do not resist it, just relax into it.

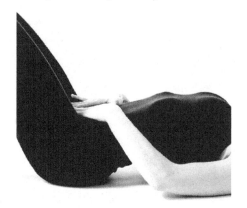

- Smoothly rock back and forth for two to three minutes to integrate Core Breathing into a bodily movement, to improve body awareness, and to increase pelvic circulation.

FROG STRETCH: This is a fantastic stretch, especially for women who experience pain or tension in the pelvic region. The "Frog Stretch" stretches and relaxes the muscles of the hips and pelvic floor.

Frog Stretch Practice:

- Lie on the floor with your hips and knees bent. Bring your legs off the floor, hold onto your inner ankles, and let your knees flop apart. Try not to allow any tension into this stretch, just pure relaxation. Feel the sensation of stretching and opening in the pelvic floor and inner thighs. Breathe deeply and relax. Hold for 30 to 60 seconds.

- Return legs to the floor, take another deep breath, and repeat (two repetitions total).

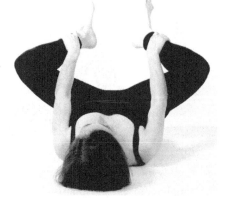

Make an effort to complete these three exercises every day as you work your way through Step One. Make it a part of your schedule, just like brushing your teeth!

Lady Bits

Goal 2: Daily Movement for Relaxation Routine

Every day, complete the following exercises. This should take no more than 7-8 minutes.

- Pelvic Drops: 5-10 repetitions
- Pelvic Rocks: 2-3 minutes
- Frog Stretch: 2 repetitions

The following is a summary of the goals for Step One. I encourage you to **master** these relaxation goals. Practice them regularly as described and turn them into habits – components of your daily routine that are as ingrained into your lifestyle as showering (you would not even consider skipping it). Your body will thank you, your mind will thank you, and you may notice that your sex life has already ramped up a notch simply because you are more able to relax and release.

Summary of relaxation goals for Step One (master these before moving on):
Goal 1: Core Breathing plus Sensual Visualization every 1-2 hours, daily
Goal 2: Complete the Movement for Relaxation routine every day

- Pelvic Drops: 5-10 repetitions
- Pelvic Rocks: 2-3 minutes
- Frog Stretch: 2 repetitions

There you have it! You have gained awareness of your inner core through a combination of breath work, visualization, movement, and stretching. You are now ready to move on to Step Two of the *Lady Bits* program... **Fitness!**

STEP TWO: TARGETED FITNESS

Now that you have integrated daily relaxation into your life, it is time to focus on strengthening, moving, and appropriately using the deep inner core muscles to awaken your (sometimes dormant) desire, and to experience the pleasure of movement...the pleasure of being in your own body. **If you haven't already sampled the Inner Core Energizer routine (Chapter 13), now is the time to start.**

We are all aware that fitness training is important for cardiovascular health, increasing and maintaining bone density, and managing weight; however, it is also important for your sexual health! The *Lady Bits* program hones in on the core muscle groups that are extremely active during sex. You will learn how to isolate these muscles, how to successfully use them during full-body activities, and how to improve overall core strength and endurance.

The following lists evidence to support inner core fitness training **specifically for enhancing your sex life**, and details the benefits you will see as you progress through Step Two:

- Regularly working the muscles of the inner core increases vascularity in the pelvic region. This **increases blood flow and circulation**. In addition, frequent practice of focused movements may stimulate nerve growth, leading to an **increase in sensitivity**. Both of these changes can **heighten sexual responsiveness and may improve libido** so that your desire for intercourse is stronger and more frequent.

- Regular strengthening will **increase muscular endurance**, which is vitally important during intimacy and in all other aspects of life.

- Understanding how to quickly and easily contract the pelvic floor before and during intercourse can **stimulate arousal**, as well as **enhance and even lengthen orgasm**.

- Inner core strengthening will **decrease problems associated with pelvic floor muscle weakness and dysfunction** such as incontinence.

- The holistic approach of combining relaxation with fitness will **improve the mind-body connection**, thereby increasing body awareness – an essential component of satisfying sex.

- There is substantial evidence to suggest that women who exercise regularly **have more energy and are happier**, two powerful aphrodisiacs.

- Regular, dedicated participation in this program will **burn calories**, allowing you to shed pounds and tone up thereby **improving body confidence**. Body confidence is positively correlated with a more active, satisfying sex life. When you feel confident about your body, you exude sexiness!

While we are on the subject of health benefits of inner core fitness, intercourse itself is an extremely healthy activity. It burns calories, releases oxytocin (the love and bonding hormone), boosts metabolism, and releases epinephrine. **Ever heard of a "runner's high?" It is comparable to the "afterglow" of sex!** In addition, regular sex can improve immune function, help you sleep better, balance your hormones, and reduce stress.

With dedication and regular practice this well-rounded program will make you feel feminine, strong, confident, and in-touch with your body (both physically and emotionally).

Goal 1: Thirty minutes of Sustained Physical Movement five days per week

Sustained Physical Movement (SPM) was discussed in Chapter 12. You can turn back to that chapter for examples, but the take-home message is that you can choose any activity you enjoy that gets your body moving and your heart rate up.

Goal 2: Complete the Inner Core Energizer three days per week

The Inner Core Energizer is detailed in Chapter 13 and video tutorials are available (for free) at www.femfusionfitness.com/energizer. Below is a summary of the routine, for your convenience. **Although the list is lengthy, remember that the exercises are meant to flow from one to the next without significant rest breaks between.**

Summary of the Inner Core Energizer:

Pelvic Rocks: 30-60 seconds

Pelvic Bounces: 30 seconds

Stirring the Pot: 5 times each direction

Open Like a Book: 3-5 times each direction

30-Second Breath Meditation

Bridge with Block into Deep Abdominal Wake-Up: 3 bridges, followed by 10 wake-ups

Long Leg Stretch: 5 times each side

V-Legs: 10 repetitions

Butterfly Bridge: 10 repetitions

*Prance into Deep Ab Blaster: 10 prances, followed by 10 blasters

Bridge with Hip Circles: 5 circles each direction

Slalom: 20 repetitions

Superwoman with Foot Taps and Mini Rear-Lifts: 3 repetitions of the entire sequence (10 foot taps and 3 rear-lifts)

Child's Pose All Directions: 15-20 seconds in each position

Kneeling Foot/Toe Stretch with Hands Clasped Overhead: 15-20 seconds

Chest Expansion: 15-20 seconds

Kundalini Heart Opener into Bust Circles: 20 heart openers, followed by 5 bust circles each direction

*Naughty Cat into Rocking Horse: 10 naughty cats in each direction, followed by 10 rocking horses on each side

Kneeling Series: 10 hip pumps, 5 hip circles each direction, 5 wide-knee kegel lifts

Side Plank with Oblique Twists: 10 twists each side

*Plank with Hip Drop: 10 hip drops each side

Downward Facing Dog with Alternating Knee Bends: 30 seconds

Pigeon Pose: 30-60 seconds each side

Deep Squat with Kegels: 30-60 seconds

Frog Squats: 10 repetitions

Hip Activator Series: 3 minutes total

Frog Squats: 10 repetitions

Standing Hip Circles: 10 circles each direction

Pelvic Roll-Ups: 10 each side

Goddess Plié Squats Into Deep Groin Stretch: 5 squats followed by 15-20 second stretch

Sexy Squats: 5 slow and sexy squats

Plié Squat with Hip Circles: Hold squat while circling hips 10 times each direction

Sunshine Breath into Forward Fold: 2 repetitions, holding the forward fold for 15-20 seconds each time

*See notes for women with diastasis recti (DR).

REMINDER: View the digital workout online at www.femfusionfitness.com/energizer.

Summary of fitness goals for Step Two:
Goal 1: Thirty minutes of SPM five days per week
Goal 2: Complete the Inner Core Energizer three days per week

You can choose whether you want to continue the daily Movement for Relaxation routine (from Step One) once you begin integrating the Inner Core Energizer into your weekly schedule. It is not required to do both, but it certainly doesn't hurt! The more movement, the better.

I do, however, encourage you to continue the Sensual Visualization from Step One. This is a great practice that can be continued indefinitely.

STEP THREE: THE CLIMAX

If you have read *Lady Bits* in its entirety, you have built a strong foundation for the best sex of your life. First you learned about your body – your unique female anatomy and physiology, the remarkable cycles that make you a woman, and the changes that are occurring (or are likely to occur) so that you can better understand and accept your body.

You began the process of creating a healthy lifestyle and radically loving yourself and the skin you're in.

You learned how to relax mind and body, and you started (and will continue) the journey toward core strength and fitness with the Inner Core Energizer routine.

Now for the climax... It's time to put it all together! In this step, I will show you how to use your newfound strength and coordination to take your intimate encounters to new heights.

Although we have touched upon sex and some other very personal subjects throughout the course of this book, you might still feel awkward reading about it. If this is a hang-up for you, please remember – sex is natural and normal. Consider:

- **We came from sex.**

- Your mother and father had sex to produce you. If they are still alive, they probably still have sex to this day.

- Most adults have sex...regularly! In fact, your co-worker may have had sex last night. Your child's kindergarten teacher probably had sex recently. Your mail carrier has sex. Just like "everybody poops," (almost) everybody has sex.

Despite a cultural undercurrent that causes many of us to subconsciously think otherwise, there is nothing dirty or shameful about intercourse. Sex and sexuality is completely acceptable when between two consenting adults. Get curious. It's okay to want to learn more about sex... It's good to be intrigued! As women, we should all strive to deeply know and understand our bodies from the inside out (which is what we've been working on since page one of *Lady Bits*), and how could this knowledge not spill over into our intimate lives?

Rather than goals, Step Three lists several techniques and ideas you can utilize before, during, and after intimacy. Step Three is a bit more involved than Steps One and Two. Don't feel like you need to sample every suggestion; take what you like, and leave the rest behind.

IMPORTANT NOTE (1): I am not a licensed sex therapist and the following information should not be considered to be therapeutic or medical advice. Please seek counseling or sex therapy from a qualified practitioner if required for your (or your partner's) specific condition.

IMPORTANT NOTE (2): Throughout this chapter I will be using the pronouns "he" and "she" when describing romantic partnerships; however, non-heterosexual readers can still utilize most of the information. Sexual preference is irrelevant when it comes to the emotional and spiritual exercises – and even some of the physical exercises – described in the following pages.

BEFORE SEX: WARM UP

Most of us idealize Hollywood romance that appears to be spontaneous and uninhibited by agenda or time. However, for many of us, intimacy might have to be scheduled. My friends anticipate the weekends that their kids sleep over at grandma and grandpa's house, or use afternoon naps as an opportunity for sex. I've had clients who have weekly "sex dates" that are so firmly planned they are written into their calendars. Some couples have sex multiple times per week, and others have sex only once every few months. Whatever your situation, and whatever your age or stage, planning is probably a reality more often than not. If so, look at it as a golden opportunity to **prepare** (both mentally and physically) so you can make the most of your intimate moments.

Without making this sound too much like spring training, I want to impart the importance of warming up before "game time." Mental and physical preparation is just as essential for you prior to sex as it is for athletes prior to a big game. As we have discussed, female brains are wired differently than male brains. Men excel at being laser-focused upon a single task. Due to tribal responsibilities of the past, women excel at having our attention in multiple places at any one time. **In order to make sex satisfying, you MUST bring your attention to the present moment.**

The first step is to mentally clear the path to romance. Take care of chores that need your attention or that seriously bother you, and then ignore the rest. Sex is not fun – and may feel like a burden – if the sink full of dirty dishes preoccupies you. If you can't stand the mess, then do the dishes (or better yet, delegate). But if you can tolerate the unsent emails or the basket of laundry waiting to be folded, wonderful. **Clear your mind of your tasks with the awareness that they can – and will – get done later.** If you have a mental "to-do" list for the rest of the day or for the following day, write it down. Do what you need to do rid your mind of excess clutter. Take a few moments to breathe deeply and center your attention on your partner and your relationship. This is where a regular practice of Core Breathing with Sensual Visualization comes in handy; think of it as foreplay that you can do all day long!

The second step is to physically warm up. Physically warming up is an important component of great sex since movement and focused attention on the pelvic region will enhance stimulation and sensitivity. The simple act of focusing your attention on any **area of the body** causes an increase in nerve and muscular activity, as well as an increase in blood and lymphatic flow. Try it now. Think about the most incredible sexual encounter you've ever had (or a fantasy you desire, that may or may not have actually occurred), and then really focus your attention on the areas of your body that felt (or would feel) "lit up" and aroused during this encounter. Feel the spreading warmth in your groin region. It might feel electric, or a little bit "buzzy," like your nerve endings are firing rapidly...because they are! **When you add physical movement such as pelvic rocks, pelvic bounces, and/or stirring the pot to these thoughts, you're literally fueling the fire in preparation for the events ahead.**

Many people do not realize that women require sufficient mental and physical arousal in order to prepare the vagina for intercourse. Arousal increases the length and caliber (internal diameter) of the vagina, so if sufficient time has not been taken to elicit arousal, your body will not be anatomically prepared for sex.

Taking the time to mentally and physically "warm up" may not always be practical or possible due to time constraints or setting. However, if you can capture a few spare moments, it will be well worth your while.

NOTE: The following routine is drawn from information already discussed. Rather than re-describe the exercises, I have referenced sections for you to refer back to if you need to refresh your memory.

EXERCISE – The Mental and Physical Warm Up:

Create a sacred, private space. What makes you feel sensual? Perhaps music, soft lighting, candles, aromatherapy or incense; whatever makes you feel comfortable, feminine, and relaxed.

Lie down in an area that is appropriate for the gentle movement routine described below. Initiate _Core Breathing (Chapter 11)_.

If time permits, complete the _Light and Love Meditation (Chapter 19)_.

Physically prepare your body for sex with the following gentle movement routine:

- _Pelvic Rocks (as described in Step One, Movement for Relaxation, and in the Inner Core Energizer)_. Focus your attention on the pelvic floor during this exercise. Feel the way your pelvic floor muscles contract gently as you press your low back into the floor. Feel the way your pelvic floor muscles relax as you gently arch the low back off the floor. This rhythmic pelvic movement pattern will increase sexual arousal.

- _Pelvic Bounces (as described in the Inner Core Energizer)_. Feel the energy gather in your pelvis and pelvic floor. This gentle exercise increases blood flow and stimulation to the pelvic region.

- _Stirring the Pot (as described in the Inner Core Energizer)_.

This flowing exercise lubricates the hip joints and stimulates the inner core muscles.

- *Frog Stretch (as described in Step One, Movement for Relaxation). This stretch relaxes the inner thigh and pelvic floor muscles, which is extremely important especially if you tend to feel tension or pain during intercourse.*

Throughout this warm up, it is essential to relax and clear the mind. If you find your mind wandering, recall your most pleasurable sexual experience, or fantasize to further facilitate arousal. Draw on your experiences with Sensual Visualization; the mental pictures you have painted with all five senses will directly impact the sexual experience for which you are preparing. Remember – focused attention and arousal (from thoughts and physical stimulation) increases blood flow to the pelvic floor and genitals. This increase in blood flow causes engorgement (swelling) of the clitoris, labia, and vagina as well as an increase in vaginal lubrication, length, and width. As you can see, warming up before game time is essential, and it can feel **really good**.

Fun Tidbit: The "Middle Way." You might notice that I've referenced Buddhist quotes and teachings several times throughout *Lady Bits*. Although I am not a Buddhist, I do identify with the Buddha's teaching of the "middle way," which – put simply – indicates living a life of moderation between two extremes. This, according to Buddha, paves the way to wisdom and happiness.

I feel that the "middle way" can be applied to many aspects of women's health and balanced, healthy living...and even to sex! **It's important to normalize expectations when it comes to what your sex life "should" look like.** In recent years popular music artists have sung about "swinging from the chandeliers" (Sia), "making love like gorillas" (Bruno Mars), and "getting your freak on" (Missy Elliot). If we are to believe romance novels, the music industry, and pop culture we would think that a sizzling sex life requires daily romps with an amazing orgasm every time. This is not reality. **If you don't want to have sex every day – or even every week – that's fine. If you like to do it in similar positions every time, that's all right, too.**

Some women DO enjoy frequent sex and "kinky" positions and scenarios, and that's wonderful! Just realize that you are not alone – and you're not a "cold fish" – if you are NOT in this subset. The "middle way" is perfectly okay.

BEFORE SEX: CULTIVATE CREATIVITY

Creativity and sex are both related to energy movement in the lower chakras (recall that chakras are energy centers in the body through which energy flows). If one aspect is flowing, the other may be more energized as well. Likewise, if one aspect is stymied – such as a busy working mom who feels like every second of her life revolves around child rearing and her job – she might begin to feel creatively frustrated, which can result in a diminished libido.

Use this awareness to spark your intimate life. In the face of sexual frustration, try being creative and see what new inspirations arise. Notice how your creative energy and your sexual energy are related. This doesn't need to take long, and it doesn't have to take the form of a masterpiece. **You can even incorporate creativity into the mental and physical warm up described above.**

EXERCISE – (Quickly) Cultivate Creativity:

Find some traditional tribal music with drums, chanting, didgeridoos, or anything that brings out the wild woman within. Anytime you have a spare moment, push play and move to the rhythm: shimmy and shake your hips, or totally let loose and dance your heart out. You can even do this with kids around, long before any intimate encounters occur. The more often you seize small opportunities for creativity, the more you'll benefit sexually.

Other ideas that you can do anytime, for as little as a few minutes a day: Write in your journal. Tackle a Pinterest project. Work on your hobby or favorite craft, add a few touches to your scrapbook, sing in the shower, draw or doodle, play the piano, draw a tasteful tattoo on your body... Be silly! Let your hair down. Try a new look with makeup. Be free... Be CREATIVE. It might spark something new in the bedroom (and beyond).

BEFORE SEX: GET (EMOTIONALLY) NAKED

Whereas men tend to think the path to emotional connection is through physicality (i.e. sex), women tend to feel the inverse: before getting physical, they need to feel mentally and emotionally secure and connected. **As a human, especially as a FEMALE human, you are wired for connection.**

When you move from a lust-based relationship (in your early months or years of dating and/or marriage) to a more established and familiar relationship, excitement wanes. **You want to be wanted the way you were when things were fresh...and you want to want them the way you did then, too!** You don't know what to do when the anticipation and lust appears to be gone. You wonder, "Is it me?" This stagnation and self-doubt can build up over time, leaving you feeling closed off and uninspired.

It's not just about the biology of getting older and the psychology of feeling more "settled" with your partner; rather, it's a lack of emotional intimacy, which can be difficult to revive without a concerted effort. You would think that the longer you've been with your partner, the easier it would be to talk about your true desires and needs when it comes to sex, but often this is not the case. It's easy to get tongue-tied, or simply to become complacent and not know how – or when – to start the conversation. You may feel vulnerable, naked, and exposed. You might be scared of rejection, confusion, or even anger.

It takes courage to be the one who softens first, especially in romantic relationships that may have experienced a build-up of metaphorical "walls" over time. **But softness, vulnerability, and increased emotional intimacy can open the door to better sex.** Throughout this book you've been working on becoming more emotionally intimate with yourself; why not bring your partner into the mix?

Be the soft, emotional, feminine woman that you are...the woman your partner craves.

The good news? **As long as you are sensitive when talking about your feelings with your partner, he is likely to be receptive.** Avoid framing the conversation in a way that implies you're disappointed with how things are now. Rather, begin with what you appreciate and enjoy in your relationship. Then dip your toe into the waters of offering suggestions for what you would like to see more of (or less of) during your intimate encounters. For example:

"I love that we've been married for 15 years and that we're so comfortable together. I feel safe asking you this because I know I can trust you... I wonder if you'd consider trying something new, sexually, with me? I'd like to mix things up a bit. I'm not bored or unhappy; I just think it would be a fun way to explore and grow together as a couple."

In this example you're emotionally undressing yourself, exposing your feelings and wishes with honesty and trust. From love and appreciation, to hesitation and concern about HIS emotions, to your desire to explore and try new things, you are being open and honest... And ultimately, that's what your partner wants.

BEFORE SEX: CLOAK YOURSELF IN CONFIDENCE

Nothing can ruin the mood faster than embarrassment, shame, and self-doubt. Many women worry that they're not "good" in bed. It might help to know that men worry about this too. The key (for both parties) is to experiment, to be open, and to communicate. Don't worry about your – or your partner's – performance. Sex isn't about the doing...it's about the being.

Even more crippling than performance anxiety is feeling ashamed of your own body. As Stefani Ruper states on her blog, www.paleoforwomen.com, "Nothing kills a libido like self-doubt."[82] If you suffer from self-doubt, I have great news for you: there is NOTHING sexier than confidence, and every woman on the planet – no matter her age, size, or body shape – has the capacity to be confident. Following the steps in this book and learning how to love, understand and accept yourself will get you there. Don't waste an ounce of thought on your squishy belly or the cellulite on your thighs. He doesn't notice; he has other things on his mind.

Think of your partner – does he always want to touch you? If so, welcome it and RECEIVE it. Feel confident in knowing that you are **worthy and deserving** of his attention and affection.

> *EXERCISE – Cloak Yourself in Confidence:*
>
> *The sexiest thing a woman can wear is confidence. Before your next sexual encounter, spend some time mentally dressing yourself in a slinky, silky, sexy negligee of self-confidence. Wrap yourself in an aura of sparkly radiance, like the stardust that encircled Cinderella as her fairy godmother used her magic wand to create her beautiful ball gown. Even if you're completely naked, you'll be fully dressed.*

In the words of women's health expert Dr. Anna Cabeca, "The number one way to turn on your man is to be turned on, lit up, and in the moment. Your turn-on is HIS turn-on."[83]

BEFORE SEX: ACCEPT CHANGES

This goes along with the previous point, but it bears repeating: dissatisfaction with your own – or your partner's – naturally aging (and changing) appearance can affect your pleasure in bed. Get over it! More likely than not, your partner doesn't notice the "flaws" that you do. If he likes what he sees, don't argue with him, and don't point out what you perceive that he "missed" or overlooked.

Physiological changes are also a typical part of aging. Take comfort in the fact that improving your level of fitness using the Inner Core Energizer routine WILL help you have better sex. In fact, a recent study in the *Journal of Sexual Medicine* showed that sexual function (including sexual desire, arousal/excitement, and orgasm) improved among women with urinary incontinence who participated in a pelvic floor strengthening program.[84]

Being physically strong and active helps you feel joy, passion, and pleasure, and allows you to get more out of life. Your radiance will shine through. People will notice. Even as your hair greys and fine lines and wrinkles set in, you will have an aura of strength, energy, and spunkiness that others will see.

Be the woman who lights up the room at twenty-five...or at eighty-five.

BEFORE SEX: SURROUND YOURSELF WITH ROMANCE

There's something to be said for romance novels, scented candles, sultry music, and all the other trappings of sensuality. Sex is big business – don't dismiss this multi-billion dollar industry!

Pop into a lingerie store and buy something lacy and seductive. Purchase a book by Nora Roberts or E. L. James. It doesn't have to be Pulitzer Prize winning literature...simply fuel for your imagination. Bringing erotic reading material into the bedroom is a great way to spark your intimate life. It can be used on your own, or it can be used as inspiration to "spice things up" if you read (or re-enact) choice scenes with your partner. Light candles or burn incense. Enjoy "setting the stage" for romance.

> **Fun Tidbit: Set the mood without polluting your body.**
> While you might be tempted by scented candles with names like "love spell" or "island sunset," many of the products you get at your local grocery or drugstore are chock-full of VOCs (volatile organic compounds), making them more polluting than soothing and romance-inducing. Many also contain phthalates, which are known endocrine disrupters. Pure, plant-derived essential oils are a great alternative. A relaxing blend for the bedroom includes lavender (which may decrease the stress hormone cortisol), roman chamomile, and ylang-ylang. Add 8 drops lavender, 3 drops chamomile, and 2 drops ylang-ylang to a one ounce spray bottle and fill the rest with water. Shake well. Spritz on bedding, draperies, and in the air. If you use candles, choose natural

beeswax or palm wax candles made with lead-free wicks and scented with pure essential oils.

BEFORE SEX: HARNESS THE POWER OF OXYTOCIN

Oxytocin is known as the "love and bonding hormone." It is released during childbirth and orgasm (among other activities), as it helps to stimulate uterine contractions. Oxytocin decreases pain, relieves stress, and improves sleep, and gives you those pleasurable warm and fuzzy feelings synonymous with holding your newborn baby or snuggling in front of the fire with your man.

Dr. Anna Cabeca, creator of the online course *Sexual CPR*, recommends cuddling with your partner for a solid two minutes before sex.[83] This serves to release oxytocin and will also stimulate the other mental and physiological responses that I referenced in the "warm up" section. Two minutes! It's not long, and can make all the difference.

Other ways to release oxytocin include hugging, kissing, laughing, playing (even with a pet), enjoying company and companionship, philanthropy, massage, and dance. Even if you don't have a romantic partner, you can still harness the power of oxytocin and enjoy its health-promoting benefits.

DURING SEX: MANTRA MAGIC

We've discussed the über-connected, always "on," multi-tasking feminine brain. Your complex neural pathways can be used to your advantage in your career and during daily tasks of living, but it can be a serious disadvantage during intimacy. Thinking of the bills, the neighbors, and tomorrow's lunch can be a real mood-killer.

Use the mantra, "I'm here now" DURING sex to keep you in the moment, and to keep your brilliant (and busy) female brain from running in 1,000 different directions.

Repeat it quietly and calmly in your mind (no need to voice it aloud). "I'm here now... I'm here now." Bring yourself fully into the moment.

Whenever your mind starts to wander, lasso it back. "I'm here now."

Whenever your thoughts start to scatter, return to the present moment. "I'm here now."

You will be amazed at how much this simple practice can help. Even better, your partner will feel your presence as well. Vietnamese monk Thich Nhat Hanh discusses "Right Mindfulness" in his book *The Heart of the Buddha's Teachings*. Granted, he is not referencing sex when he states the following, but it can absolutely be applied to lovemaking (as well as all other aspects of relationship): "To love means to nourish the other with appropriate attention. When you practice Right Mindfulness, you make yourself and the other person present at the same time."[85]

Once you STOP being mentally dispersed, you can be truly present. And when you're present, you not only gift yourself the full experience of being in the moment, you also gift your partner with your full attention. He can feel it, and he will flourish under it.

DURING SEX: THE CHAKRA DANCE

Throughout *Lady Bits*, I have referred to chakras and energy. As I move through my own healing journey, I have found that practices related to keeping my life-force energy balanced and clear and keeping my chakras glowing brightly are foundational to health, happiness, unabashed femininity, and uninhibited love and intimacy.

Although I am still a beginner when it comes to studying and working with my chakras, I can guarantee that if you are open to learning about the chakra system, your life will open up in more ways than one. It took me several years to really "jump in" to this subject matter, but once I did...wow.

There are seven chakras in your body. Chakras are loci of energy, or "wheels of light" (in Sanskrit) that interact with specific endocrine glands by feeding in good energy and disposing of unwanted energy. The base or "root" chakra (Muladhara) is the first chakra. It interacts with the testes in males and the ovaries in females, and is typically associated with the color red. The sacral chakra (Svadisthana) is the second chakra. It interacts with the adrenal glands and is typically associated with the color orange. Moving up your spine (and up the line of chakras) you have your solar plexus chakra (associated with the pancreas and the color yellow), heart chakra (associated with the thymus and the color green), throat chakra (associated with the thyroid and parathyroid glands and the color blue), brow or "third eye" chakra (associated with the pituitary gland and the color indigo), and the crown chakra (associated with the pineal gland and associated with the color violet).[86]

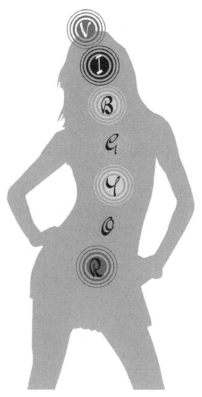

Remember the acronym ROY G. BIV? It's not only a way to remember the sequence of hues that make up a rainbow, it's also a way to remember your chakras: red, orange, yellow, green, blue, indigo, and violet. For a full-color download of the following graphic, go to www. femfusionfitness.com/images.

ROY G. BIV mnemonic for the chakras

If you choose to study the chakra system, you will learn how to sense and activate each of your chakras. You might notice energetic blocks in certain chakras, which indicates stagnation or stasis. **Keeping your chakras clean, clear, and glowing brightly can play a major role in sex and intimacy as well as general health.** In relation to intimacy, the first two chakras are your sexual and sensual centers, connected with your basic impulses, instincts, and vitality. The third and fourth chakras correlate with self-worth, self-confidence, love, and connection.

As you learn how to activate you chakras on your own, you might find that this ability spills over into the bedroom. One of the most magical experiences you can have is to sense and activate your chakras during sex. Light them up, one by one, with your strongest energetic focus on your first and second chakras. Sense wheels of red and orange light in your pelvic region, and feel these wheels of light glowing and overflowing into your partner. You might sense his chakras lighting up, as well. The mind-body sensation of these energetic centers merging, and increasing in power and intensity as you and your partner connect, is exhilarating... potent...intoxicating. I call it the "chakra dance," and it's something I recommend you try.

Medical intuitive Belinda Davidson's work is an excellent resource for learning and understanding the chakra system (www.belindadavidson. com). See the Resources section for more information.

DURING SEX: USING KEGELS TO ENHANCE INTIMACY

Other than being in the moment, the key to stimulating sex is **rhythm**. With or without kegels, sex is a rhythmic activity with motions and sensations that occur quickly, slowly, and everything in between. To add to this cadence, contract your pelvic floor muscles rhythmically to help build your arousal toward orgasm.

Contraction of the pelvic floor muscles increases blood flow to the pelvic and vaginal regions, which increases arousal and lubrication. The "warm up" (described above) starts this process by gently moving, stretching, and using the deep core muscles. Continue moving, gently contracting, and fully relaxing the muscles during foreplay in order to further increase pelvic arousal and stimulation.

The following techniques utilize the inner core coordination you have gained over the last few weeks of practice DURING SEX. These are not "one size fits all" suggestions; depending on your level of pelvic floor muscle strength, endurance, and coordination, some techniques may work better for you than others. Experiment, communicate with your partner, and see what feels best to you.

Kegels During Sex:

- **Quickies:** Have your partner enter and linger inside of you for a few moments. Before he withdraws, rapidly contract your pelvic floor muscles once or twice. Repeat as often as desired.

- **Slow and Steady:** Hold a gentle pelvic floor muscle contraction (kegel) for as long as possible while making love, and then fully release. Feel the sensation of your muscles in a fully relaxed state, then contract and hold again. Repeat as often as desired.

- **Tight Entrance:** Contract your pelvic floor muscles as your partner enters, and relax your pelvic floor as he withdraws.

- **Don't Let Go:** Relax your pelvic floor muscles completely (you can even bear down **very gently**) as your partner enters, and then complete a strong kegel as he withdraws.

- **Complete Surrender:** Fully relax your pelvic floor muscles and **very, very gently** bear down for 10-15 seconds. Totally release, get still, and just ENJOY the sensations. Please note that the very gentle "bearing down" is simply a **complete release** of the pelvic floor muscles. It should not feel like a "push."

- **Surprise:** Intersperse periods of pelvic floor contraction and periods of pelvic floor relaxation throughout the sexual experience. Spend a few minutes without doing kegels at all, and then do any combination of the above suggestions for 30 to 60 seconds. Mix it up!

Have fun with this! Take turns with your partner; follow his lead in terms of speed and intensity, then have him follow yours. There are just two important things to remember: keep your contractions rhythmic, and remember that relaxation is just as important as contraction. **This isn't meant to be labor-intensive or thought-intensive.** If you get tired, take a break!

Do not feel ashamed or embarrassed if your partner does not feel your pelvic floor muscle contractions. Your muscles may not be strong enough for him to sense a strong grip, or he may be so lost in the myriad of sexual sensations that he does not register the stimulus you are providing. Kegels during intercourse are primarily for **you**. They may (or may not) stimulate your partner but in the context of this book, your partner's stimulation is not the primary goal. Although intercourse is all about sharing and experiencing together, the techniques described in this program are ultimately for you and your own personal pleasure.

DURING SEX: KEGELS DURING ORGASM (EXTRA CREDIT KEGELS)

Female orgasm is traditionally defined as "the pleasurable contraction of the pelvic floor muscles, and the smooth muscle of the vagina and uterus."[87] If you have experienced orgasm (keep in mind, not every woman has), you will recognize the pulsing sensation that occurs in the pelvic region when you climax. This feeling – often described as "wave-like" or even "electric" – is the sensation of a buildup of muscular tension that is involuntarily released by orgasm. Deliberately completing *extra* pelvic floor contractions (kegels) is like doing **extra credit**, utilizing your inner core muscles to push you above and beyond. "Extra credit kegels," as I like to call them, can help you reach climax, can intensify the experience, and can make your orgasm last longer.

Here is how you can deepen your experience of climax by completing extra credit kegels: as you feel your pelvic floor muscles naturally begin to pulse, **add to the intensity of the contractions with your own deliberate kegels**. Work with your body's own speed. If your body pulses quickly, add to the orgasmic pulses with intentional quick kegels. If you feel slow, languid pulsing, complete your kegels more slowly. Work with the rhythm of your own body.

As mentioned above, some women have never experienced orgasm. This is not uncommon – if you are anorgasmic, you are not alone and you are certainly not "frigid" or any other condescending, old-fashioned term that still circulates in our culture. According to the authors of *Becoming Orgasmic*, "About 15 to 20 percent of the cases seen in sex therapy involve women who have never experienced orgasm. An even greater percentage of cases involve women who are orgasmic but who experience difficulty reaching orgasm."[88] Dr. Anna Cabeca reports that 80% of women have difficulty achieving orgasm from vaginal intercourse alone, and she encourages women to re-define "orgasm" as the ENTIRE EXPERIENCE of sex, not just the climax.[83]

If you have difficulty reaching orgasm and have not experimented with mechanical stimulation, consider purchasing a small vibrator that you can use – very gently – on your clitoris. As mentioned in Chapter 5, the clitoris is an extremely sensitive area that is much larger than it appears. The small area of tissue you can see and feel at the top of the vagina is just the apex of a huge network of nerves that travel along both sides of the vagina beneath the labia. Find a comfortable, quiet, private spot to use your vibrator and see what happens. If you are sufficiently relaxed, you may experience a clitoral orgasm and will sense the pulsing sensations described above. Once you are comfortable experiencing these sensations, enhance your experience with the extra credit kegels discussed above.

If you still cannot elicit orgasm (and if you wish to), please refer to the Resources section at the end of this book for a list of books and websites with information you may find helpful. Orgasmic Meditation, in which sexual intercourse is not even involved, can be a wonderful way to elicit orgasm via a process of deep relaxation and clitoral stimulation.[89] If you haven't experienced it, I encourage you to give it a try.

Some women are able to experience a different type of orgasm – a "deep pelvic orgasm," or "expanded orgasm." During a deep pelvic orgasm, instead of the pelvic floor rhythmically contracting, the pelvic floor muscles actually relax and the deepest, most interior aspect of the vagina tightens. As stated in *The Multi-Orgasmic Woman*, "although some women have these orgasms spontaneously, most women need to be taught to access their potential for deep pelvic orgasm... It is experienced more by releasing and less by grasping."[87] The authors state that **the key is to fully relax**, let go of any mental resistance to fully experiencing the orgasm, and to allow yourself to **gently push out** with your pelvic musculature (in other words, fully relax your pelvic floor). Emptying the bowels or bladder before intercourse can help with fears about accidents, since gently pushing out and relaxing the pelvic floor muscles can be associated with elimination.

To be clear, deep pelvic orgasms are associated with pelvic floor muscle relaxation and release. If you wish to experiment with deep pelvic orgasms, do not complete extra credit kegels during the orgasm; rather, focus on kegels **leading up to** the orgasm or possibly completing kegels **after** the orgasm to extend the pleasurable sensations (see the following section).

DURING SEX: EXTENDING ORGASM

In addition to leading up to climax and intensifying orgasm, additional pelvic floor muscle contractions **after orgasm** can make the waves of pleasure last longer. Try extending your orgasm by doing kegels continually, even after the sensations of climax have subsided. As stated in *The Multi-Orgasmic Woman*, by doing so, "you are consciously continuing and encouraging pulsations, and as you train your body, you will find that you can keep the pleasurable waves coming."[87]

To practice this technique, follow your body's lead and maintain your personal cadence of rhythmic pulsing after orgasm. Try to move continuously from orgasm to voluntary pelvic floor muscle contraction without much of a break. For example, as you orgasm, add to the pulsing sensation with your own deliberate kegels as described above in the section titled "extra credit kegels," then – seamlessly, without skipping a beat – **continue to rhythmically contract your pelvic floor after your body's natural pulsing subsides**.

Extending orgasm with kegels does not work for everyone. Some women are simply too tired to elicit additional muscular contractions after they climax. Experiment, and see what works best for you. Try not to take things too seriously, and try not to "over think" the situation! Always remember to be gentle with yourself, and be patient. Remember, practice makes perfect.

DURING SEX: POSITION CONSIDERATIONS

I wish I could recommend a **magic position** that would enhance every woman's sexual experience, every time. But the reality is that every woman's preferences are different and every woman's anatomy is slightly different. The position of your pelvic organs and the angle and length of your vagina varies throughout your lifetime – even throughout your monthly cycle. In addition, as we've discussed, vaginal tissue integrity changes after childbirth (vaginal deliveries can cause scarring and stretching) and as you age (tissues tend to thin as estrogen levels decrease). Most significantly, personal preference varies wildly! As a general rule, work with a position that makes you comfortable. If you are not flexible, having sex while attempting to do the splits will not work for you. You will be so focused on the discomfort of the position that you will not be able to relax and concentrate on what feels good.

When experimenting with positions, always consider your personal resting level of pelvic floor muscle tension. By this point in your journey toward inner core health and wellness, you should have a good internal sense of your pelvic floor musculature. Do your muscles tend to be tense? Do you have a hard time relaxing after you complete a kegel? Do you tend to be constipated? Do you ever have pain during or after intercourse, during or after a bowel movement, or during tampon insertion? Do you have problems with urinary frequency? These are some common signs that you might have hyperactive – or overly tense – pelvic floor muscles. If this is the case for you, I recommend sexual positions that allow you to fully relax; for example, lying on your back (with your partner in the "missionary position") or lying on your side. Some women with tense pelvic floor muscles do well on their hands and knees, or resting on their elbows and their knees (which causes the hips to be elevated above the shoulders and slightly stretches the muscles of the pelvic floor). When lying on your back you might try putting a pillow under your hips; this allows you to relax, but also puts you in a good position to stimulate the G-spot and the AFE (anterior fornix erogenous) zone – two sensitive areas that can elicit orgasm in many women.

If the questions above do not apply to you and if you feel that you are able to contract and relax your pelvic floor muscles freely, then you will likely be comfortable in any position. Being on top increases control, which many women enjoy. It allows you to direct the speed, intensity, and angle of penetration. However, being on top does require more muscular activation, which is why this position should be avoided – at least initially – if your pelvic floor muscles tend to be tense or hyperactive. With awareness of personal pelvic floor muscle activity level and focused relaxation training (which often requires help from a specialist such as a psychologist or a women's health physical therapist), women who have a history of pelvic floor muscle hyperactivity can learn how to relax their pelvic floor muscles and gradually switch to more active positions.

The other factor to consider when thinking of sexual positions is your personal level of pelvic floor muscle strength. If you plan complete kegels during sex, you need to be strong enough to contract the muscles against gravity if you prefer to be on top. If you are strong enough to easily contract and relax your pelvic floor muscles while sitting or standing, you are ready for more upright sexual positions. If you are not yet able to easily contract and relax your pelvic floor muscles while sitting or standing, it will be most effective for you to do kegels in sexual positions that do **not** require you to move your pelvic floor muscles against gravity. Kegels are easiest when lying down on your back, lying on your side, or lying with your hips propped up on pillows; thus, these types of sexual positions are optimal when you are building pelvic floor muscle strength.

Of course, when experimenting with any new position, remember to start slowly and gently. **If something does not work for you, just laugh it off and move on.** Feeling comfortable in your own skin allows you to dismiss things that don't work with grace and poise... *and nothing is sexier than confidence!*

LOOKING AHEAD: KEEP IT SPICY

Boredom is one of the biggest risks of a sustained monogamous relationship, so talking openly about sex, trying new practices (such as

Orgasmic Meditation), adding new "moves" (such as the kegels described in this book), experimenting with lights (on versus off), taking it to different rooms or locations, and making love at different times of the day are all simple ways to mix things up and keep the spark alive. Keep in mind that if you have children, this can be EASIER as the kids get older and more independent. There is no reason to think that sex and sexuality must decrease with age. You actually have a lot to look forward to!

All this being said, there is no shame in keeping things simple and basic. Everyone is different, and there is no single "right" way to enjoy intimacy.

LOOKING AHEAD: OPEN UP AND LIGHTEN UP

Couples can fall out of their normal sexual patterns for any number of reasons, and once this happens, it can be difficult to get back on track. The longer the break, the harder it can be to start up again. A decrease (or even cessation) of sexual activity can become the proverbial "elephant in the room;" something that both of you think about, but neither brings up as you settle into bed for the evening. What to do in this situation? Talk about it! Having a sense of humor can help, and being brave and vulnerable enough to be the one to bring it up is essential.

Furthermore, it's not uncommon for men to develop sexual difficulties as they age. Erectile dysfunction (ED) is incredibly common, and between not being able to "get it up," not being able to "keep it up," premature ejaculation, or – at the other extreme – taking too long to ejaculate, the entire topic of sex has the potential for discomfort and awkwardness. Don't let it get that way. Keep it light. Seek help from a qualified sex therapist if needed, and most importantly...just RELAX. Anxiety and stress are often the primary contributors to not only the female's difficulties with sex, but the male's difficulties as well.

PART VII:
Making The Change

INFORMATION WITHOUT ACTION
IS JUST MIND CLUTTER.

*"Sometimes it's the smallest decisions that can
change your life forever."*
–Keri Russell

*"If you're waiting to 'never be scared' to take action you're never going to
get anywhere, because part of growing is
getting out of your comfort zone."*
–Jessica Ortner

*"You must live in the present, launch yourself on every wave,
find your eternity in each moment. Fools stand on their island
of opportunities and look toward another land.
There is no other land; there is no other life but this."*
–Henry David Thoreau

.

Chapter 22

PUTTING IT ALL TOGETHER
(BRINGING *LADY BITS* TO YOUR REAL LIFE)

You understand your body, you know what you need to do to take care of yourself, and you know the steps to sizzling sex. Now let's bring *Lady Bits* into YOUR reality, and really make a change!

We have already established that you can't fit into someone else's box when it comes to healthy living; everyone is biologically different (bioindividuality), the structure of everyone's lives is different, and everyone's goals and dreams are different. **In order to make the *Lady Bits* three-step system work for you, you need to make it personal.**

THE SHOULD SHOW

I consider "should" to be a dirty word. It immediately makes me feel contracted and anxious. If I "should" be doing something, it means that I'm not doing it now, which implies negativity, badness, and shame.

I first heard the term "the should show," from Jessie May, a life coach with an inspirational self-help podcast called *Sunny Side Up*. Jessie equates "should" to shame, a word that can make you feel "less than" and disempowered. She talks about "shoulding all over the place" (which always makes me laugh), and Lord knows I've spent most of my life doing that! How about you?

If you tend to "should all over the place," it's time to clean it up.
All it takes is a simple switch from the word "should" to the words "choose to." Let's take fitness as an example, which is – of course – a significant theme of this book. As you begin to make healthy changes in your life, rather than think, "I should exercise more," think to yourself, "I choose to exercise more."

Instead of "I should lose this weight," think, "I choose to lose this weight."

Instead of "I should have sex with my husband tonight," think, "I choose to have sex with my husband tonight."

What a simple but powerful shift! For me, when I change my verbiage from "should" to "choose to," I immediately feel expansive, powerful, and motivated rather than contracted, inadequate, and less-than.

VISION: WHAT DO YOU WANT MOST?

This is the fun part – getting clear on what makes you feel good; what feels like a "hell YES!" in your body, mind, and soul. As I stated above, everyone's goals and dreams are different. **So... What is the outcome YOU most want to obtain?**

You have to know what you're running toward before you can figure out how to get there.

EXERCISE – Visioning:

Really think about your personal "hell YES!" vision. What do you hope to achieve after you've started – and stuck to – the Lady Bits program? A more sensual, exciting relationship with your husband? A toned, lean body? More confidence? More energy? More self-love? A better relationship with yourself?

Grab a piece of paper or your journal, and write down your vision – that which feels like a resounding "yes" in your body. Now take a minute to really consider something. Do you want this particular outcome for the right reason?

If your perspective isn't right, you are likely to fail. Your reason(s) for change must be intrinsic; something you would do if you were stranded on a deserted island and there was no one there to "look good for," or to do it for. Something you would do **no matter what**, simply because you want to do it for YOU.

- Losing ten pounds because your doctor "said so" isn't for YOU, it's for your doc!

- Dropping a dress size before your twenty-year high school reunion to make your former rival jealous isn't for YOU; rather, it's an "eat your heart out" declaration that's directed externally.

Why are you expending the energy to make these healthy changes? This is your time to be selfish; it's the only way to make changes that will last. **What's in it for YOU?**

Here are some subtle shifts that can change the above (extrinsically directed) examples into intrinsic visions:

- Losing ten pounds in order to feel energetic and vibrant, and to live a longer life, so you can spend more time with your family and friends.

- Dropping a dress size in order to feel confident and secure, knowing that you've blossomed into a beautiful, strong woman over the last twenty years.

Continuing with the visioning exercise, write 1-3 reasons why you want to turn your vision into a reality. Make sure the reasons for change are for YOU (intrinsic), and not for anyone else.

In order to be successful with this program you're going to have to get clear on WHY you're participating so that you can have something to draw upon when all you want to do is stay in bed, watch re-runs of Friends, and drink hot chocolate.

FEEL THE FEELINGS BEHIND YOUR VISION

Next, spend a few minutes visualizing the FEELING(S) you wish to achieve. Not so much the vision you identified above; rather, the **feelings** behind your vision. You can begin visualizing (and feeling) immediately... even before you've started to take action.

As Mike Dooley, author of *Infinite Possibilities*, states: "Thoughts become things."[90] But emotions and feelings are even **stronger** than thoughts when you visualize. Emotions and feelings are the true drivers of transformation when it comes to manifesting change in your life!

Take the time to complete this exercise. It really is a game-changer.

> *EXERCISE – Feel the Feelings:*
>
> *Remind yourself of your vision and write it down again (refer to the previous page).*
>
> *Remind yourself of the 1-3 reasons WHY you want to turn your vision into a reality (again, refer to the previous page). I know, I know...this is redundant! But writing things over and over is good for making ideas "stick."*
>
> *Now identify 3-5 FEELINGS that you will feel once you have achieved your vision, and write them down.*

I like examples. If you do too, try this on for size:

Jackie's vision is to lose the last stubborn 10 pounds.

Jackie's (intrinsic) reasons for change are:

- She wants to **feel good** in her favorite pair of jeans.
- She knows that she'll have **more energy** when she's carrying less weight. More energy will help Jackie be able to do more of the things that she wants to do in life.
- She wants to **set a positive example** for her friends and family. Being a leader motivates Jackie to keep going. She likes the feeling of being the one that people look to for guidance.

The FEELINGS that Jackie will feel when she loses the excess weight: **radiance, ease, happiness, vibrancy, pride, and confidence**.

So when she visualizes each evening before bed, Jackie will visualize the following:

- How RADIANT and SVELTE she'll feel in her clothes.

- The EASE she'll feel, being able to slip on her favorite pair of jeans without having to tug, cinch, or suck in.

- How HAPPY, ENERGETIC, and VIBRANT she'll feel as she plays with her kids, and how good she'll feel about being able to keep up with them.

- How PROUD she'll feel when her friend notices a change but can't quite identify it (*"You look different...in a good way!"* her friend will say, and Jackie will beam with pride).

- How CONFIDENT she'll feel at her next office party, KNOWING that she looks as good as she feels.

NOTE: When you visualize yourself feeling these wonderful feelings – already having reached your target outcome or vision – don't worry about HOW you're going to get there. Try NOT to think about the journey and the twists and turns along the way. Visualization time is not a time for planning, scheming, or scheduling. It's a time for seeing – in your mind's eye – the desired outcome and FEELING the feelings as if you have already reached your goal(s).

Feel the feelings and emotions you will feel when you're "there." See yourself THERE. Feel yourself THERE. Weave stories and daydreams of what life will look like when you're THERE. This process gets you in touch with your deepest desires; the only true driving force when it comes to making positive, lasting change. **This is powerful stuff!**

WILLPOWER

The word "willpower" is laden with pressure, expectation, and emotion. The word itself implies that if you have the power to stick to your will, then you're strong; you've succeeded. If you don't have the power to stick to your will, you're weak; you've failed.

Keep in mind that willpower is a limited resource. Big goals and broad, sweeping changes are difficult – if not impossible – for most people to make (and keep) all at once. **Small changes are ideal, as is finding a way to be "consistently consistent."** Although DESIRE and VISION drive change on an emotional and spiritual level, consistency is what ultimately makes change happen on a physical level.

Overly ambitious goals can set you up for stress and "yo-yo" performance (as in overly restrictive dieting or daily participation in a grueling fitness program). Progress, not perfection, is the key to reaching your goals: lots of small changes that build up over time. It's easy to get caught up in an "all or nothing" mentality, and then when you can't (or don't) give it your all, you stop.

> **Remember: No matter how many times you fail, course-correct, or fall short of your goal...**
>
> **Keep showing up.**
> **You will screw up.**
> **That doesn't mean you should GIVE UP.**

When life throws you a curveball and you don't get all of your workouts in, you get too busy to prepare "clean" meals and snacks in advance, or you don't get enough sleep one night, don't worry. **All is not lost.** Stay positive and think about all that you have accomplished toward your healthy living goals, and commit to making the next day just a little bit better.

Don't wait until you reach your goal to be proud of yourself. Be proud of yourself every step of the way. Keep showing up! **It's not about willpower, it's about consistency.**

> **"Life always offers you a second chance...**
> **It's called TOMORROW."**
> **–Author Unknown**

Chapter 23

DO YOU HAVE TIME TO FEEL BAD?

If you want to make healthy changes but you haven't, and you're justifying your stagnation to a lack of time, then take a step back to really evaluate your situation. As one of my spiritual mentors, Gabrielle Bernstein, says: "Do you have time to feel like crap?" Think about it. Just a few minutes out of your day could change your life.

"Just a few minutes a day? Everything you've talked about would take HOURS!"

I want to make this crystal clear: **you do not need to adopt all of the lifestyle changes that I've described in this book, nor do you have to make all of the changes all at once**. Furthermore, you certainly do not need to tick off every suggestion in Step Three of the *Lady Bits* three-step system for better sex. If you did, you wouldn't have time to work or even to sleep! Choose what resonates with you – the practices that will best help you embrace your femininity, inhabit your body, and honor your sexuality. Think of these as your launching points.

TIME MANAGEMENT

The most common complaint I hear among women who want to adopt a healthier lifestyle – but don't – is that they do not have sufficient time to fit exercise and self-care into their daily schedules. I understand. I am a working mother – writing, developing and teaching fitness classes, and promoting my business. I also cook three meals a day, tend to our home, shuttle my son to and from school and extracurricular activities, and try to keep up with blog entries and social networking. I do my best to carve out sufficient time for my friends and (of course) my family. Sometimes I can do it all...and as I've related several times throughout this book, sometimes I feel a bit frazzled. When I start feeling frazzled – or if my health begins to suffer – I've learned to take a step back and see what needs to be changed.

> **"When it is obvious that the goals cannot be reached, don't adjust the goals, adjust the action steps."**
> **–Confucius**

Women often feel inadequate, messy, tired, and sometimes a little insane. Their self-esteem takes a wallop every time they get pumped up for change but then fall off-track due to life's (many) curveballs. In order to reverse the shame we might feel when this happens, we can (and must) align reality with expectations of how life "should" be.

It's easy to think, "I should be able to get all this done," when the reality is that it's just not possible to do it all, all at once. As women, we tend to put everyone else's needs ahead of our own, and that's got to stop. **To adopt a healthier lifestyle, you're going to have to prioritize, plan, (likely) ELIMINATE, and seek support.**

The fact that you purchased this book indicates that you are interested in changing something about your current level of health and wellness so do not allow yourself the "I should, but…" or the, "I want to, but…" or the, "I just don't have the time" excuses. That is all they are: excuses. Saying or thinking them will not change anything. They will not magically give you more time, they will not make you fitter, they will not improve your sex life…they won't even make you feel better (instead, you'll just feel stuck). **So, please, skip the excuses and just get started.** Remember, it's not that we "should" do this, it's that we CHOOSE to do this.

I apologize in advance for the language, but this quote is so fitting for the subject at-hand:

> **"I've never seen any life transformation that didn't begin with the person in question finally getting tired of their own bullshit."**
> **–Elizabeth Gilbert**

Here are some suggestions for carving out extra time for relaxation, exercise, and clean eating (because let's face it, it does take more time and energy to cook and shop for clean meals than to purchase take-out). Pick one or two ideas to begin, and watch time expand!

First, some fantastic tips from the FemFusion community:

- *"Vastly limit the time that is spent watching TV and get up one hour earlier than everyone else in the house."*

- *"I spend a couple of hours every Sunday prepping food for the week. I make a big batch of soup and that's my lunch for days. Also, when I get together with friends I try to plan something active for us to do (paddleboard yoga, indoor rock climbing, pole class) so I'm getting a 'girl date' and a workout at the same time."*

- *"Freezer meals. I'm just getting into this... I prepped twelve meals at the beginning of the month and haven't had to ask, 'what's for dinner' once! It's given me a little more wiggle room to exercise in the afternoons when I would have been cooking."*

- *"I started with a ten-minute daily exercise goal. It felt manageable, and although my goal is seven days a week, I am happy with five days. I focus on HIIT (high intensity interval training) and light weight training. I now have the energy and motivation to get up 30-45 earlier than my early risers."*

- *"I wash all my fruits and veggies as soon as they come in the door, and meal plan for at least a week at a time."*

- *"Look at your daily chores. Many of them can be done every-other-day (rather than every day) and many can also be consolidated. Now that I'm retired my issue is no longer about time, it's more about smart energy expenditure. I'd rather bike than vacuum, or dig in the garden versus mop the floor."*

Now, some suggestions from me:

- **Plan your next day the night before.** It's so much easier to show up for yourself when you know where you're supposed to be! Prioritize and allot time for each task by blocking it out in your daily planner, and then stick to your schedule. Fluidity is okay, but it is important to start with – and commit to – a plan. If an unexpected appointment comes up during your workout time, simply move your workout to later in the day (or earlier). But don't blow it off! You wouldn't blow off a business meeting or medical appointment; don't blow off your health goals, either.

- **If you're more of a week-at-a-time planner, consider creating a "Time Map."** See Appendix B for a Time Map template. Look at your calendar for an average week and then block off all time that is UNAVAILABLE to work on your health goals. Mark out time spent sleeping, time spent getting ready to leave the house in the morning, work, time spent driving to/from work and/or driving your kids to activities, scheduled social activities, food preparation (and eating), wind-down time before bed...even shower time! **Be specific. This allows you to take a realistic look at the time you have LEFT OVER to work on the *Lady Bits* program.** You might want to exercise first thing every morning as recommended in the forthcoming 14-Day Action Guide... But do you actually have time to do that? The Time Map can help you figure it out. Based on the (realistic) weekly snapshot that your Time Map provides, adjust your priorities and commitments accordingly so that you have time to work on your health goals.

- **Make a "hell no" list and let go of what you don't want. This is important – probably the most important tip in this list.** You can't just keep putting things on your plate; in order to make sustainable change, you're going to have to take something off. Through the process of identifying your "hell yes!" vision in Chapter 22, you can now clearly identify the things that you do NOT want in your life...the activities that are crowding out your (extremely limited) resources of time and energy. What tasks, commitments, and responsibilities contribute to stress, overwhelm, and anxiety? It is essential to really take a step back and look at your life and what's working for you – and what's not – so that you can make positive changes, and ultimately, be happy! As business coach Marie Forleo says, "If it's not a hell yes, then it's a hell no." **Come up with activities that support your "hell yes" vision, and let go of as many "hell no" activities as possible.** Do you really want to be the mom who makes snacks for your son's soccer games, or can someone else take care of it? Are you still benefiting from the foreign language class you're taking? How about that work committee you volunteered for? Weigh the costs and benefits of the extraneous activities in your life and gracefully exit the ones that no longer serve you. It can be brutal, but you must find a way to free up your valuable time.

- **Figure out the timing that works best for YOU.** For me, morning is "magic time." As Louise Hay states, "How you start your day is how you live your day," and I couldn't agree more. **Try it for yourself: take advantage of the morning's peace and quiet and challenge yourself to wake up 30 minutes earlier than you normally would. Use this time to work on the** Lady Bits **program, daily meditation and relaxation, or healthy meal preparation.** However, everyone is different. If you already know that mornings are "out," don't force yourself out of your comfort zone and into mine. If you fight yourself every step of the way, you're not going to stick with it. If you are a night owl, dedicate 30 minutes of quiet time in the evening to healthy living practices rather than television, social media, or work.

- **Ask for (and accept) help.** Your family might not do things as thoroughly or as well as you, but by asking them to help with the laundry or the errands, or by asking a friend to watch your child for an hour each week, you'll be able to carve out more time for yourself and your goals. Explain to your husband that you are trying to create more time to exercise in order to enhance your sexual health and see how quickly he helps out with dishes or gets the kids to sweep the floor!

- **Be obvious.** Leave yourself gentle – but clear – cues that simply cannot be missed. Leave your yoga mat unrolled on the living room floor so that it's waiting for you in the morning. Place your walking/running sneakers right in front of the door. Place your healthiest food and snack options front and center in your fridge or cupboard. As I like to say, "You've got to make the right thing to do the easy thing to do."

- **Break up your exercise sessions.** Some days you might have an uninterrupted hour to dedicate to SPM, whereas other days you might perceive no time at all. Challenge this perception... I'll bet you have time to fit a few mini exercise sessions into your day. The following routine takes five minutes flat: 15 push-ups, 15 squats, 15 lunges, and a 30-60 second plank. Do it. Right now! Don't you feel better? Sneak that into your day three times and you'll be set. You can even close your office door and do it at work.

- **Walk during part of your lunch break.**

- **Exercise or focus on your relaxation techniques during your child's nap/quiet time, or while watching his/her sports practices or games.**

- **Cut down on tech time.** The Internet has become an integral part of daily life and spending time on the computer (or other technological device) is a necessity for many people. However – admit it – we also waste a lot of time online. A 2014 article from TechCrunch.com reported that American Facebook users spend around 40 minutes each day using the service, an astonishing 1200 minutes per month.[91] And Facebook is **just one** of the many social networking sites that people frequent! You could spend that time sitting on your duff catching up with people you hardly know/ barely remember, or you could invest that time in your health. Leave Facebook for the weekends or cut down your usage to just five minutes per day for a quick status update and a brief check on essential people and pages. Substitute exercise time for Facebook (or Instagram or Pinterest, etc.) time and see how much better you feel.

- **If you want to take this a step further, consider a "digital detox."** Take three to four days completely OFF of technology. It will be hard but you might realize that it was making you unhappier and less connected rather than happier and more connected.

- **Zen your inbox.** Email unsubscribe services (such as www. unroll.me) are available – often free of charge – and can help you declutter your inbox by allowing you to unsubscribe from multiple email lists all at once. This is a simple way to save time and energy. If it no longer serves you, unsubscribe. A clean, streamlined inbox is incredibly calming.

- **Dust off your slow cooker.** Throw some meat and veggies in the slow cooker in the morning and exercise during (what would normally be) dinner preparation time in the early evening.

- **If you have the financial means, hire someone to take on some of your tasks.** Sign up for a grocery delivery service, or hire a housekeeper. This will allow you more time to focus on learning how to make some of the healthy changes I've described WITHOUT feeling like you are neglecting the maintenance of your home or pantry. If you run a business, hire a three to four hour per week employee (college students are great for this) to complete routine tasks that can be delegated. I actually hired my friend's ten-year-old son to make some simple changes on my website. Today's kids are often more tech-savvy than we are!

- **Above all, remember flexibility, balance, and the 80/20 Rule (Chapter 16).** Life happens. Things will come up. That doesn't mean you should give up!

In short, please do not use the "I don't have time" excuse unless you've exhausted the tips in the list above, paying special attention to the tip about ELIMINATING as many "hell no" activities as possible. Chances are there is a spot somewhere in your life that has the potential to be used for your health goals rather than tasks or commitments that no longer serve you. Your energy level, confidence, and **happiness** depend on it.

DRAINERS VERSUS FILLERS

As holistic nutritionist Leanne Vogel states, "There are people in your life that suck you dry. And, there are people that fill you up. Defining which is which will literally set you free."[92]

EXERCISE – Compile a "Drainers" Versus "Fillers" List:

Consider your friends, co-workers, family members, and other social circles (even online communities) and list who fills you up, and who drains you. Drainers can be thought of as "energy vampires," people who – possibly for reasons you can't even identify – make you feel tired, contracted, or bogged down when you are in their presence (or soon after you've left them). Don't feel vicious for doing this activity... just be honest! It might surprise you who comes to mind as a drainer. Do you naturally surround yourself with negativity?

The key is to limit time spent with people who bring you down, and spend more time with people who make you FEEL GOOD. Start asking yourself, "Who fills me up? And how can I act so that I may be a 'filler' as well?"

Another key is to surround yourself with people who are in your corner and who are living their own vision. This will help you see what's possible! Beware, you might need to seek new social connections as you begin to make healthy lifestyle changes. Everybody needs someone to believe in them; unfortunately, this doesn't always come in the form of your close family or friends. You might need to hire a coach or healer, or find a support group, fitness class, or other healthy living resource (live or online). Find a tribe of women who understand and can connect with what you're going through. You are much more likely to make changes that last when you have support...when you're not going it alone.

"You are the average of the five people you spendthe most time with."
–Jim Rohn

One of my clients, Kay, was doing a great job of "cleaning up" her family's diet. Kay's family doctor wanted her daughters to start eating gluten-free for medical reasons. Her family was doing well and felt fantastic, but a certain friend kept making mean-spirited remarks, completely sabotaging Kay and undermining her efforts. Kay didn't understand it. This individual had been a family friend for years!

I helped Kay realize that often, these individuals are scared or threatened when they see you making positive changes that they either don't understand, or that they might not be able – or willing – to keep up with themselves. They see the changes as a threat, and ultimately, they're scared they're going to lose you. So they have a choice: to rise to your level, or to knock you down...and frankly, it's easier to knock you down. They probably don't even know they're doing it...but if they are, you need to distance yourself and choose peers who will support you and lift you up instead. This is NOT a simple task, but it's essential to your success.

> "Surround yourself with people who make you happy. People who make you laugh, who help you when you're in need. People who genuinely care. They are the ones worth keeping in your life. Everyone else is just passing through."
> –Karl Marx

PROTECT YOURSELF: THE SENTRY GODDESS

You have identified your VISION, and you've actively felt the feelings behind it. How are you going to make sure that life doesn't encroach on your plans for health and personal growth? You must be flexible enough to accept that things won't go exactly as planned. But on the other hand, there are plenty of invasions of your time and energy that you have control over. **Your task is to decide what information, opportunities, interactions, and tasks you're going to let into your life, and what (and who) you are going to keep out.**

I've already referred to your "hell no" tasks/activities and social "drainers." You need to be leery of these invaders. What you need is a sentry to keep watch over you: someone (or something) to protect both you and your vision.

Exercise – The Sentry Goddess:

When I want to protect a new habit that I'm trying to cultivate, or a new direction that I'm trying to grow (because we are so tender when changes are fresh!), I use a tool that I've dubbed my "sentry goddess." I call upon my "sentry goddess" to protect the seeds of change that are growing within me. You might want to try this too.

I imagine a small garden near my third chakra, the energy center associated with self-worth, motivation, energy, and achievement. The third chakra is located in the solar plexus, just under the sternum (breastbone). My imaginary garden is delicate; the little seeds are just starting to sprout. There's a fence around my garden, with a gate. The gate can be opened to let in information, tasks, people, and activities that I choose – but it can also be closed and locked.

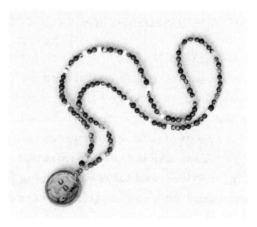

My "sentry goddess" necklace

It is helpful for me to have a physical reminder that I don't have to let everything into my garden – that I don't have to say "yes" to all opportunities, I don't have to listen to every bit of information or piece of advice that comes my way, and I don't have to accept every single responsibility. I created a "sentry goddess" to guard my imaginary garden gate by purchasing a small indulgence: a delicate mala bead necklace with a pendant of a beautiful goddess that dangles right between my breasts, at my solar plexus chakra (the very chakra that needs protection and support when making changes). I wear this necklace almost every day as a reminder of the goddess within me – the "sentry goddess" who guards my garden gate. She is always looking out, deciding who and what she'll let in, and when.

LADIES, LET'S DO THIS

Making healthy changes can be challenging, and let's face it, quitting has become a bad habit for many of us. You must learn to get comfortable with discomfort when shifting to a healthier lifestyle. Keep in mind that understanding your body, knowing and loving your body, and learning how to properly care for it is an investment in your health – an investment in yourself. And it's one of the most lucrative investments you'll EVER make.

> **"No one is in control of your happiness but you; therefore, you have the power to change anything about yourself or your life that you want to change."**
> **–Barbara De Angelis**

Lady Bits is just like any other fitness and lifestyle program in that **consistency is key**. You will not see a change if you use this information once and then forget about it. Regular practice will pull your focus inward, cultivating your feminine energy and strengthening your inner core…the very center of your femininity.

The program found in this book is complete – it encompasses much more than doing a few kegels each day. As you have seen, *Lady Bits* focuses on improving your overall health; mind, body, and spirit. The Inner Core Energizer **utilizes all of the muscles of the inner core** rather than relying on kegels alone to rev up your sex drive, improve stability, and increase bodily control.

Building upon the foundation of knowledge you accumulated in the first five parts of this book, I introduced the *Lady Bits* three steps to better sex program in Part VI.

- Step One taught you how to relax deeply and easily, and how to enjoy foreplay throughout the day (Sensual Visualization).

- Step Two showed you how to use targeted core fitness to strengthen your core and bring pleasure back into your body.

- Step Three listed suggestions for actions to take before, during, and after sex. Consider this the icing on the spiced-up sex life cake.

My sincere hope is that the exercises and lifestyle implementations found in this book have helped you feel stronger, more feminine, and more confident than ever before. There is nothing sexier than that!

Chapter 24

YOUR DAILY ACTION GUIDE:
A 14-DAY PLAN

Information without action is just mind clutter...so take some action.

True, 14 days isn't long enough to create a true transformation, but it's short enough to "stick to" and long enough to show you just how good you can feel making these simple lifestyle shifts. Give the *Lady Bits* program your all for two weeks and see how radiant you can feel, at any age.

The *Lady Bits* program is not a magic bullet or a quick fix – you will not notice any changes if you do not **commit** to practicing the steps described in this book, and outlined below in the 14-Day Action Guide.

You will not gain strength immediately; in fact, it takes weeks for muscles to hypertrophy (gain mass) and increase endurance. What you **will** notice almost immediately is the effect of concentration and focus on the muscles of the inner core. Within just a few days of practice, you will note changes in sensation, tone, and activity level of the inner core muscles simply from neuromuscular reeducation, or the mind-body connection that allows you to "re-learn" how to use certain muscle groups. If you have never worked your deep core muscles before, you may feel some initial muscle soreness. This will pass. If you note soreness or strain that does not pass or in fact worsens, please consult your physical therapist, physician, or other qualified healthcare provider. If you have any questions based on your specific medical needs, please check with your healthcare provider before beginning the 14-Day Action Guide.

If you prefer to do things on your own, here is a reiteration of the *Lady Bits* program:

- Understand your beautiful, unique female body and take baby steps toward improving your health using the information gleaned from Parts I through V.

- Move on to the **Three Steps to Better Sex System** detailed in Part VI.

- **Step One:*** Complete the Movement for Relaxation routine every evening to prepare your mind and body for Steps Two and Three.
Enjoy Sensual Visualization daily.

- **Step Two:** Complete the Inner Core Energizer routine three times per week.
Enjoy 30 minutes of SPM five days per week.

- **Step Three:** Spice up your sex life with any (or all) of the suggestions listed.

*NOTE: Step One is meant to prepare your mind and body for Steps Two and Three. You do not need to continue the Movement for Relaxation routine and Sensual Visualization breaks indefinitely – you might only need them for a few days or even a week to get the ball rolling and your juices flowing. That being said, you are welcome to continue with them long-term. They are easy to integrate into your daily routine and regular relaxation practice will help you handle the trials and tribulations of everyday life with grace.

If you like a done-for-you plan, then the following 14-Day Action Guide is for you. It incorporates the relaxation techniques from Step One as well as the fitness plan from Step Two. It also incorporates some of the lifestyle strategies referred to throughout the earlier portions of the book, from self-love techniques, to rest and relaxation, to eating clean.

Remember, this 14-Day Action Guide is just a suggestion. It's quite fluid, and not at all rigid or restrictive. Feel free to modify this plan as needed to fit your personal needs and lifestyle.

Day 1 – Monday:

- First thing in the morning, wake up and enjoy a large glass (12-16 ounces) of lukewarm or room temperate water to hydrate your body and stimulate your digestive system. Move your body in a way that feels GOOD. Stretch, do some hip circles, and take deep, cleansing breaths.

- Move more throughout the day. Enjoy a 30-minute walk with friends (or alone) on your lunch break.

- At least once today, try Sensual Visualization (Chapter 21).

- Before bed, complete the Movement for Relaxation exercises (Chapter 21), and the Light and Love Meditation (Chapter 19).

Day 2 – Tuesday:

- First thing in the morning, wake up and enjoy a large glass of lukewarm or room temperate water. Move your body in a way that feels GOOD. Stretch, do some hip circles, and take deep, cleansing breaths.

- Continue to move more throughout the day. Change positions as often as possible (alternate between sitting and standing). Take a few minutes to do 15 push-ups, 15 squats, and 15 lunges at least three times today, and try to sneak in a 15-minute walk before or after work.

- At least three times, take 60 seconds for Sensual Visualization. Use a sticky note or alarm to remind you to take these breaks.

- Before bed, complete the Movement for Relaxation exercises and the Light and Love Meditation.

Day 3 – Wednesday:

- First thing in the morning, wake up and enjoy a large glass of lukewarm or room temperate water. Move your body in a way that feels GOOD. Stretch, do some hip circles, and take deep, cleansing breaths.

- Before work, complete the 25-minute Inner Core Energizer routine.

- At least three times during your workday, take 2-3 minutes for Sensual Visualization. Use a sticky note or alarm to remind you to take these breaks.

- Before bed, complete the Light and Love Meditation.

Day 4 – Thursday:

- First thing in the morning, wake up and enjoy a large glass of lukewarm or room temperate water. Move your body in a way that feels GOOD. Stretch, do some hip circles, and take deep, cleansing breaths.

- Focus on incorporating Sensual Visualization into your day more often, with the goal of 60 seconds of Sensual Visualization every one to two hours. You may want to use a sticky note or alarm to remind you to take these breaks.

- Move more throughout the day. Enjoy a 30-minute walk with your friends (or alone) on your lunch break. Take 5 minutes to do 15 push-ups, 15 squats, and 15 lunges at least once today.

- Before bed, complete the Movement for Relaxation exercises.

Day 5 – Friday:

- First thing in the morning, wake up and enjoy a large glass of lukewarm or room temperate water. Move your body in a way that feels GOOD. Stretch, do some hip circles, and take deep, cleansing breaths.

- Before work, complete the 25-minute Inner Core Energizer routine.

- Focus on incorporating Sensual Visualization into your day with the goal of 60 seconds of Sensual Visualization every one to two hours.

- Make a list of five reasons why you love yourself, and post it somewhere you'll see. Consider copying this list two or three

times, and place copies of the list in various places throughout
your home or office so that it catches you off guard – in a good
way – whenever you glimpse it.

- Before bed, complete the Light and Love Meditation.

Day 6 – Saturday:

- First thing in the morning, wake up and enjoy a large glass of
  lukewarm or room temperate water. Move your body in a way
  that feels GOOD. Stretch, do some hip circles, and take deep,
  cleansing breaths.

- Try something new. Seek out a 60-minute yoga class (look for a
  "beginner" class if you're new to the practice).

- Today, challenge yourself to disconnect from all technology and
  be present with what's happening right in front of you rather than
  what's going on in the digital world. This is especially important if
  you identify as an introvert or an empath (Chapter 9).

- Before bed, complete the Light and Love Meditation.

Day 7 – Sunday:

- First thing in the morning, wake up and enjoy a large glass of
  lukewarm or room temperate water. Move your body in a way
  that feels GOOD. Stretch, do some hip circles, and take deep,
  cleansing breaths.

- Complete the 25-minute Inner Core Energizer routine and follow
  up with a vigorous 30-minute walk.

- Meal plan for the week ahead. Create a grocery list and stick to
  it when you're at the store. Cook a large batch of soup (using
  nourishing bone broth as a base). Soup is on the menu for dinner
  tonight, and leftovers can be used for your lunch for the next few
  days. Reference Chapter 14 for more on clean eating.

- Before bed, spend a few moments in gratitude for your
  successful week.

Day 8 – Monday:

- First thing in the morning, wake up and enjoy a large glass of lukewarm or room temperate water. Move your body in a way that feels GOOD. Stretch, do some hip circles, and take deep, cleansing breaths.

- Look at yourself in the mirror and say, "I love you (insert name)." Do you mean what you say? If you don't, try it again. Reference Chapter 19 for more on mirror work.

- Move more throughout the day. Enjoy a 30-minute walk with friends (or alone) on your lunch break.

- Before bed, complete the Light and Love Meditation.

Day 9 – Tuesday:

- First thing in the morning, wake up and enjoy a large glass of lukewarm or room temperate water. Move your body in a way that feels GOOD. Stretch, do some hip circles, and take deep, cleansing breaths.

- When you dress for work today, wear something racy underneath your clothes. Put on your sexiest bra, your laciest panties, or take a few minutes to paint your nails a rich, luxurious red. Unleash your inner goddess.

- Again, focus on incorporating Sensual Visualization into your day. Aim for 60 seconds of Sensual Visualization with Core Breathing every one to two hours throughout the day.

- After work, complete the 25-minute Inner Core Energizer routine. Consider whether you prefer exercising in the morning or in the evening, and adjust your schedule (and the remainder of this Action Guide) accordingly.

- Before bed, complete the Light and Love Meditation.

Day 10 – Wednesday:

- First thing in the morning, wake up and enjoy a large glass of lukewarm or room temperate water. Move your body in a way that feels GOOD. Stretch, do some hip circles, and take deep, cleansing breaths.

- Before work, enjoy a vigorous 30-minute walk.

- At lunch, eat mindfully. Sit comfortably (at a table) and take a moment to look at your food BEFORE diving in. Breathe calmly and deeply as you appreciate the effort that went into making your meal, the colors of the food and the different textures and shapes... Appreciate the way it's going to nourish your body and keep you satisfied until your next meal. Bless your food with: "Thank you for the energy you bring me. Thank you for the nourishment you provide. Thank you for the pleasure you impart." And then SAVOR. Even if it's not the "perfect" meal, health-wise, when you eat with stress or fear it's going to eliminate any bit of goodness there would have been otherwise. In summary: Stop, sit, appreciate, and ENJOY.

- Before bed, complete the Light and Love Meditation.

Day 11 – Thursday:

- First thing in the morning, wake up and enjoy a large glass of lukewarm or room temperate water. Move your body in a way that feels GOOD. Stretch, do some hip circles, and take deep, cleansing breaths.

- Before work, complete the 25-minute Inner Core Energizer routine.

- Move more throughout the day. Take 5 minutes to do 15 push-ups, 15 squats, and 15 lunges at least twice today. Remember the 30-30 Rule (Chapter 9), especially if you have back or neck pain.

- Light a candle and listen to relaxing music when cooking and eating your dinner this evening.

- Before bed, complete the Light and Love Meditation or Sensual Visualization.

Day 12 – Friday:

- First thing in the morning, wake up and enjoy a large glass of lukewarm or room temperate water. Move your body in a way that feels GOOD. Stretch, do some hip circles, and take deep, cleansing breaths.

- Having lunch with your friends? Walk to meet them. Enjoy a 15-minute walk to the restaurant, and a 15-minute walk back to work (or home).

- If you struggle with body image issues, ask yourself the following questions: How do you want to be known? How do you want to be remembered? Is it your looks or size, or it is the ways in which you contribute to the world? Make a list of the positive ways you do (and will) contribute to the world, and note the most – if not all – of these things have NOTHING to do with your physical appearance. Post this list somewhere you can see it.

- Before bed, complete the Light and Love Meditation or Sensual Visualization.

Day 13 – Saturday:

- First thing in the morning, wake up and enjoy a large glass of lukewarm or room temperate water. Move your body in a way that feels GOOD. Stretch, do some hip circles, and take deep, cleansing breaths.

- Did you like last week's yoga class? If so, do it again. If not, try something new. Go golfing, play tennis, go for a swim, putter in the garden, try a new fitness class, or go dancing this evening. Spice it up!

- When you're out and about, keep your eyes (and heart and mind) open to the women around you. Notice the beauty in every shape and size, not just society's ideal of "perfection." Challenge your own beliefs about what you think is beautiful.

- Before bed, complete the Light and Love Meditation or Sensual Visualization.

Day 14 – Sunday:

- First thing in the morning, wake up and enjoy a large glass of lukewarm or room temperate water. Move your body in a way that feels GOOD. Stretch, do some hip circles, and take deep, cleansing breaths.

- Complete the 25-minute Inner Core Energizer routine and follow up with a vigorous 30-minute walk.

- Meal plan for the week ahead. Create a "clean" grocery list and stick to it when you're at the store. Double-up on tonight's healthy dinner so that you have leftovers for lunch tomorrow. If you have time, make additional meal(s) you can freeze for later.

- Before bed, spend a few moments in gratitude for your successful week.

LADY BITS LONG-TERM

You've got the foundation, and now you have a 14-day blueprint for success when it comes to loving your body, caring for yourself, living a healthier life, and having satisfying (dare I say amazing?) sex.

But true success, lasting change, and long-term results come only when you no longer need the blueprint. That's when you know you have transformed: when you are ready to toss the formula and roll on your own... That's when you know you've "got it."

It's like learning how to cook. At first, you follow recipes to the letter because you need to know the basic steps, the guidelines for combining flavors, and the science of how ingredients interact with one another. Cooking is all about trial and error. You will make mistakes, you'll develop personal preferences, and slowly – over time – you'll discover your OWN way of doing things.

No one steps into the kitchen an immediate "Master Chef." But as you get more comfortable in the kitchen, you start playing around and you intuitively "know" how to make a recipe your own. You might add a pinch of cayenne to really kick up the flavor, or you might eliminate the mushrooms because they're just not your thing.

The same goes for this program. Think of the steps in this book – and the 14-Day Action Guide provided – as jumping-off points that you can use to make a lifestyle recipe that's completely and uniquely your own.

Try it, flow with it, see how you like it, take what you love and leave the rest behind.

Just like you may never be a James Beard Foundation Award-winning chef, you may never fully "get there" when it comes to your health journey. However, you can darn well feel better and better as you immerse yourself in the process of ARRIVING. Stay humble, stay open, and stay curious. There's always more to learn and there's always room to grow. **In the space between, enjoy the ride.**

A LIFETIME OF BENEFITS

You have reached the conclusion of *Lady Bits*! How do you feel? I hope that you feel sexier, more confident, more in-tune with your body, and stronger than ever before. By completing this program, you have:

- Gained an increased awareness of your unique female anatomy and physiology.
- Learned the importance of strengthening and caring for your deep, hidden inner core muscles with fitness routines you can use for life.
- Understood the value of healthy living when it comes to healthy aging and long-term wellness.
- Learned how to love and accept yourself FIRST.
- Learned how to clear space and time for self-love and relaxation...two essential components of mental and physical health AND a rockin' love life.
- Reclaimed your radiance, your desire, and your sexual spark.

This is a comprehensive lifestyle guide with a focus on whole-woman wellness (mind, body, and spirit), but we spent a significant amount of time focusing on core fitness. And for good reason! The inner core keeps you balanced, strong, and pain free; it provides the foundation for trunk stability and is the key to bodily confidence and control.

While they are not "glamour muscles" like six-pack abs and bulging biceps, **the inner core muscles should not be a source of shame or embarrassment**. Just like our "lady bits," we need to talk about the inner core – particularly the pelvic floor – with our daughters, our mothers, and our friends. We need to make sure our fitness instructors are aware of the inner core muscles and the importance of activating them regularly and effectively.

It is time to take the taboo and the mystery out of female anatomy, sexuality, and inner core fitness. These subjects are not "icky," "dirty," or intended only for the pleasure and enjoyment of others. Yes, enhancing intimacy is the focus of this book, but above and beyond great sex is the mind-body connection I hope you have created with the deep, female center of yourself.

By understanding and appreciating your body, toning up with the Inner Core Energizer, and actually making some of the changes described in this book, you will improve your overall body confidence and allow yourself to fully **shine**. And that, my friends, is the embodiment of SEXY.

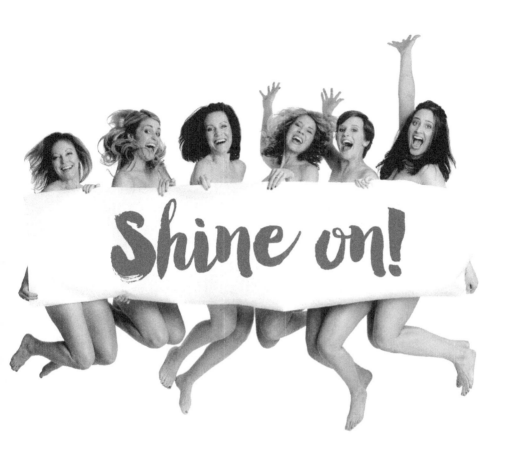

Appendix A: Period, Mood, and Moon Tracker

Downloadable at www.femfusionfitness.com/images © *Lady Bits*, 2015

Menstrual Marker	Date	Mood/ Other	Moon Phase
First day of period			
Day 2			
Day 3			
Day 4			
Day 5			
Day 6			
Day 7			
Day 8			
Day 9			
Day 10			
Day 11			
Day 12			
Day 13			
Ovulation*			
Day 15			
Day 16			
Day 17			
Day 18			
Day 19			
Day 20			

Day 21			
Day 22			
Day 23			
Day 24			
Day 25			
Day 26			
Day 27			
First day of period*			
(flex room)			
(flex room)			

*These are approximations based on an average 28-day menstrual cycle. Your cycle might be slightly different.

Directions: Use this chart to track your next menstrual cycle so that you can begin to make correlations between your changing hormone levels, your mood, and the cyclical rhythm of the natural world. **Begin on the first day of your next menstrual period (i.e. the day you begin bleeding).** In the second column, record the date. In the third column, record your mood and/or motivation as you noted it throughout the day. You can also record anything notable in relation to your creativity, energy, and/or sensations of womb energy – see Chapter 5 ("Womb Power"). In the far right column, track the moon phase. Go outside and take a look, then record an approximation of the moon phase (i.e. new, quarter, half, or full). You can also use a moon phase calendar to see the exact phase relative to your hemisphere. Example of an online resource: www.moonconnection.com.

Appendix B: Time Map

Downloadable at www.femfusionfitness.com/images

	MONDAY	TUESDAY	WEDNESDAY	THURSDAY	FRIDAY	SATURDAY	SUNDAY
12:00 AM							
1:00 AM							
2:00 AM							
3:00 AM							
4:00 AM							
5:00 AM							
6:00 AM							
7:00 AM							
8:00 AM							
9:00 AM							
10:00 AM							
11:00 AM							
12:00 PM							
1:00 PM							
2:00 PM							
3:00 PM							
4:00 PM							
5:00 PM							
6:00 PM							
7:00 PM							
8:00 PM							
9:00 PM							
10:00 PM							
11:00 PM							

TIME MAP PURPOSE: To determine your available time to work on health and self-care goals each week (i.e. fitness, meditation).
TIME MAP TECHNIQUE: Using the schedule above, block off time where you are sleeping, driving, working, have appointments, taking care of children, meal/prep eating, personal care (i.e. showering!), or any other obligations. Be realistic, and be complete! The time that is "left over" or unaccounted for can be used for your health and self-care goals.
Note: Time Map exercise inspired by **BizChix.com**

© Lady Bits, 2015

RESOURCES FOR HEALTHY LIVING AND FURTHER LEARNING:

The following books, programs, providers, and retail products are based on my personal research, preferences, and/or experience. This resource list is provided for your convenience only; it is not to be seen as an endorsement or guarantee of usefulness or availability of any particular product or provider. There are no affiliate links listed below.

As of this writing, all books and retail products are widely available in public libraries and/or online stores (such as www.amazon.com) unless a specific web address is referenced. **Internet addresses are accurate as of April 15, 2015.**

ADVANCED TRAINING FOR HEALTH AND FITNESS PROFESSIONALS:

- The Integrative Pelvic Health Institute (www. integrativepelvichealthinstitute.com) founded by Jessica Drummond, MPT, CCN, CHC is an excellent resource for professionals interested in pursuing advanced training and/or careers related to women's health and nutrition coaching.
- Burrell Education (www.burrelleducation.com) founded by Jenny Burrell, BSc offers high-quality programs, trainings, and events – both live and online – geared toward fitness professionals and healthcare providers who work with women. A special emphasis is placed on the needs of antenatal and postnatal clients.

ADRENAL FATIGUE:

- *Rethinking Fatigue: What Your Adrenals Are Really Telling You and What You Can Do About It* (e-book), by Nora Gedgaudas, CNS, CNT, available online at www.primalbody-primalmind.com/rethinking-fatigue
- *The Hormone Cure: Reclaim Balance, Sleep, Sex Drive, and Vitality Naturally with The Gottfried Protocol*, by Sarah Gottfried, MD

ANATOMY:

- For realistic 3-D video tutorials, check out www.anatomyzone.com.
- The informational site www.3dvulva.com "helps men and women

visualize and understand female reproductive and sexual anatomy."
It is an educational site – not an erotic site – and I feel that it
should be required reading for females in high school-level sexual
education classes and beyond.

- The Beautiful Cervix Project at www.beautifulcervix.com
encourages women to learn cervical self-exam and fertility
awareness in order to promote body confidence and health.

AUTOIMMUNITY:

- *The Paleo Approach: Reverse Autoimmune Disease and Heal Your Body,*
by Sarah Ballantyne, PhD

BODY IMAGE:

- Dr. Joy Jacobs is a clinical psychologist who specializes in the
treatment of children, teens and adults with eating disorders and
body image concerns (www.drjoyjacobs.com).

- Isabel Foxen Duke is a trail-blazing health coach who helps women
"stop feeling crazy around food." Private coaching options are
available, and she offers free resources at www.isabelfoxenduke.
com.

- The National Eating Disorders Association (NEDA) offers a toll-free
helpline available to help you in assessing options for yourself or a
loved one who may be struggling with an eating disorder. Call the
helpline at (800) 931-2237.

- *Over The Moon* is an online magazine (and podcast) featuring
a variety of topics related to women's health, body image,
spirituality, the Divine Feminine, and so much more... Visit www.
overthemoonmag.com.

- *Love Your Body: Positive Affirmation Treatments for Loving and
Appreciating Your Body,* by Louise Hay

ENERGETIC AWARENESS AND HEALING:

- *Wild Creative: Igniting Your Passion and Potential in Work, Home, and
Life,* by Tami Lynn Kent

- *Wild Feminine: Finding Power, Spirit, and Joy in the Female Body*, by Tami Lynn Kent

- Belinda Davidson is a medical intuitive, teacher, and healer. She offers several free resources including a chakra cleansing kit and weekly white light healings at www.belindadavidson.com.

EMOTIONAL FREEDOM TECHNIQUE (TAPPING):

- *The Tapping Solution: A Revolutionary System for Stress-Free Living*, by Nick Ortner

- *The Tapping Solution for Weight Loss & Body Confidence: A Woman's Guide to Stressing Less, Weighing Less, and Loving More*, by Jessica Ortner

FITNESS AND YOGA:

- FemFusion® Fitness... But of course! Visit me at www.femfusionfitness.com.

- Nia® is a sensory-based movement program I have experienced for myself; it is a fitness class unlike any other. Learn more at www.nianow.com.

- S Factor™ is a fitness technique that "teaches women the language of their bodies through fluid feminine movement" (www.sfactor.com). Live classes are offered, as well as DVD instruction for distance learning. I also recommend the book, *The S Factor: Strip Workouts for Every Woman*, by founder Sheila Kelley.

- For fantastic free online yoga videos, check out www.bemoreyogic.com.

GUIDED MEDITATION, VISUALIZATION, AND RELAXATION:

- *Living Goddess Meditation*, by Jon Gabriel (audio program) can be purchased at www.thegabrielmethod.com/store.

- *Heart Beats: Music-Infused Insights*, by Monique Rhodes (audio program)

MINDFULNESS:

- *The Heart of the Buddha's Teaching: Transforming Suffering into Peace,*

Joy, and Liberation, by Thich Nhat Hanh

- *Mindfulness Meditation: Nine Guided Practices to Awaken Presence and Open Your Heart*, by Tara Brach

- NON-TOXIC BEAUTY AND SKINCARE:

- *Absolute Beauty: Radiant Skin and Inner Harmony Through the Ancient Secrets of Ayurveda*, by Pratima Raichur and Mariam Cohn

- Primal Pit Paste™ (available at www.primalpitpaste.com) is a pure, non-toxic deodorant that I use on a daily basis. Other natural beauty and skincare products are available from Primal Products LLC, including lip balm, body butter, and even dental care.

- The wildly popular blog www.wellnessmama.com is a treasure-trove of information related to non-toxic living, including natural beauty and skincare recipes you can make in your kitchen.

NUTRITION AND DIET:

- *Sexy by Nature: The Whole Foods Solution to Radiant Health, Life-Long Sex Appeal, and Soaring Confidence*, by Stefani Ruper. This book is truly a must-read and a book that belongs in every woman's library.

- *The Slow Down Diet: Eating for Pleasure, Energy, and Weight Loss*, by Marc David

- *Happy Belly: A Woman's Guide to Feeling Vibrant, Light, and Balanced*, by Nadya Andreeva

- *The Unconventional Weight Loss Convention*, hosted by Suz Crawt. Audio recordings can be purchased at www.unconventionalweightloss.com/order/.

A SELECTION OF MY FAVORITE COOKBOOKS:

- *The Longevity Kitchen: Satisfying, Big-Flavor Recipes Featuring the Top 16 Age-Busting Power Foods*, by Rebecca Katz and Mat Edelson. Note: This cookbook utilizes more grains and legumes than I typically eat, but it's vegetable-centric (which I appreciate), and the flavors are incredible. The "Kitchen Pharmacy" section was used as a reference for my "Lusty Lady Smoothie."

- *The Fresh Energy Cookbook: Detox Recipes to Supercharge your Life*, by Natalia Rose and Doris Choi

- *Mediterranean Paleo Cooking: Over 150 Fresh Coastal Recipes for a Relaxed, Gluten-Free Lifestyle*, by Caitlin Weeks, Nabil Boumrar, and Diane Sanfilippo

- *Everyday Paleo Thai Cuisine: Authentic Recipes Made Gluten-Free*, by Sarah Fragoso

- *Practical Paleo: A Customized Approach to Health and a Whole-Foods Lifestyle*, by Diane Sanfilippo

- *The 21-Day Sugar Detox: Bust Sugar and Carb Cravings Naturally*, and *The 21-Day Sugar Detox Cookbook: Over 100 Recipes for Any Program Level*, both by Diane Sanfilippo

A SAFE, FOOD-BASED CLEANSE:

- *The Weekend Reboot* digital e-course, available at www.weekendreboot.com

PELVIC PAIN AND DYSPAREUNIA:

- *Heal Pelvic Pain: The Proven Stretching, Strengthening, and Nutrition Program for Relieving Pain, Incontinence, IBS, and Other Symptoms*, by Amy Stein, MPT

- *A Headache in the Pelvis (Expanded 6th Edition): A New Understanding and Treatment for Chronic Pelvic Pain Syndrome*, by David Wise, PhD & Rodney Anderson, MD

- The American Physical Therapy Association's Section on Women's Health has a great website for medical providers as well as patients, including a PT locator (www.womenshealthapta.org).

- The National Vulvodynia Association (www.nva.org) can help you learn more about vulvar pain. The site has plenty of free information for both health professionals and patients.

PREGNANCY, POSTPARTUM, AND PARENTING:

- *Hab-it Pelvic Floor: Exercises to Combat Prolapse* is an instructional program created by physical therapist and women's health expert Tasha Mulligan (www.hab-it.com). Mulligan also offers a series of exercises designed specifically for pregnancy at www.hab-it.com/videos-preg.html.

- *MuTu® System* is a "complete body make-over for moms" with a special emphasis on postpartum solutions for diastasis recti and pelvic floor weakness. Online videos and programs available at www.mutusystem.com.

- *Baby Bod: A Groundbreaking Self-Care Program for Pregnant and Postpartum Women*, by Marianne Ryan, PT

- *Reviving Your Sex Life After Childbirth: Your Guide to Pain-free and Pleasurable Sex After the Baby*, by Kathe Wallace, PT

- It's so great I just have to list it again... The blog www.wellnessmama.com is a must-peruse for all women. Katie, the founder of Wellness Mama, is a wealth of knowledge when it comes to healthy and natural living, natural pregnancy and birth, positive parenting, and more.

SELF-CARE, SELF-PRESERVATION, AND PERSONAL DEVELOPMENT:

- *The Art of Extreme Self-Care: Transform Your Life One Month at a Time*, by Cheryl Richardson

- *Infinite Possibilities: The Art of Living Your Dreams*, by Mike Dooley

- *You Can Heal Your Life*, by Louise Hay

- *Radical Acceptance: Embracing Your Life With the Heart of a Buddha*, by Tara Brach

- *The Gifts of Imperfection: Let Go of Who You Think You're Supposed to Be and Embrace Who You Are*, by Brené Brown

- *Thrive: The Third Metric to Redefining Success and Creating a Life of Well-Being, Wisdom, and Wonder*, by Arianna Huffington

- *Quiet: The Power of Introverts in a World That Can't Stop Talking*, by Susan Cain

- *The Wellness Wonderland Radio with Katie Dalebout* is one of my favorite podcasts; it is accessible at www.thewellnesswonderland. com.

- *Awaken Radio with Connie Chapman* is another inspiring podcast I enjoy. Listen at www.conniechapman.com/awaken-radio.

SEX AND SEXUALITY:

- *Slow Sex: The Art and Craft of the Female Orgasm*, by Nicole Daedone

- *The Multi-Orgasmic Woman*, by Mantak Chia & Rachel Carlton-Abrams, MD

- *Becoming Orgasmic*, by Julia Heiman, PhD & Joseph LoPiccolo, PhD

- Dr. Anna Cabeca's online course, *Sexual CPR*, is a resource to help you learn more about how specific hormonal imbalances can impact your sexual health (and so much more)... Learn more at www.sexualcpr.com.

WOMEN'S HEALTH:

- *The Wisdom of Menopause: Creating Physical and Emotional Health During the Change*, by Christiane Northrup, MD

- *Women's Bodies, Women's Wisdom: Creating Physical and Emotional Health and Healing*, by Christiane Northrup, MD

- *The Hormone Cure: Reclaim Balance, Sleep, Sex Drive, and Vitality Naturally with The Gottfried Protocol*, by Sarah Gottfried, MD

- The Women's Health Foundation (www.womenshealthfoundation. org) is home to a community blog that can be browsed by life stage, from the teen years through menopause. Content is regularly updated.

- The American Congress of Obstetricians and Gynecologists (www. acog.org) can help you locate an Ob-Gyn in your area and reports current information and research related to women's health.

- Jane Appleyard is a Chartered Physiotherapist based in the United Kingdom who works with women all over the world via her groundbreaking website, www.stressfreewoman.com. Jane offers online consultations for women with pelvic floor concerns such as incontinence, prolapse, and sexual dysfunction.

- Want to do more with your kegels? Elvie is a new kind of wearable technology; it is a biofeedback device with sensors that connect to an app on your device (phone or tablet) that guides, corrects, and visualizes your kegel exercises in real-time. Available for order at www.elvie.com.

- Michelle Lyons' website, www.celebratemuliebrity.com, features an integrative approach to women's health with content for female patients and women's health practitioners alike.

MY DISTANCE HEALERS (SERVICES AVAILABLE ONLINE):

- Lisa Finchum is a health coach, certified Reiki practitioner, certified Emotion Code practitioner, and psychic medium. She is totally approachable and a true light in the world of health and healing. Lisa offers sessions in-person and online at www. hopeholistichealth.com.

- Danielle Paige is an intuitive astrologer and healer whose work gave me clarity and focus for the "next steps" on my own health and healing journey. Learn more at www.healingpaige.com.

My website, www.femfusionfitness.com, is a resource for information, inspiration and encouragement related to all manner of women's health and fitness-related topics. I welcome your visit!

REFERENCES

NOTE: Every effort was taken to provide sufficient information for you to be able to access and obtain the original sources referenced in *Lady Bits*. In my research, I used a combination of print materials (books and peer-reviewed journals) as well as online resources (periodicals, web-based trainings and interviews, and blogs/websites belonging to experts in their field and credible associations). In some instances, I was unable to locate specific authors and dates of publication. For that reason, (n.d.) = no date. DOI provided when available. **All Web addresses valid as of April 15, 2015.**

1. Davies, M (2014, Sept 1). Just HALF of women can locate the vagina on a diagram of the female reproductive system. *MailOnline*. Retrieved from http://www.dailymail.co.uk/health/article-2739552/Just-HALF-women-locate-vagina-diagram-female-reproductive-system.html

2. Moran C, Lee C (2014). What's normal? Influencing women's perceptions of normal genitalia: an experiment involving exposure to modified and nonmodified images. *BJOG, 121*(6), 761–766.

3. Kent, T (2014). *Wild Creative: Igniting Your Passion and Potential in Work, Home, and Life*. Hillsboro, OR: Beyond Words.

4. Ovaries. (n.d.). In *You & Your Hormones, Society for Endocrinology* online website. Retrieved from http://www.yourhormones.info/glands/ovaries.aspx.

5. Drummond, J. (2014). *Your Cycle and Your Life: A Monthly Map for Moms* [PDF document]. Retrieved from the Integrative Pelvic Health Institute member portal (IPHI students only): http://integrativepelvichealthinstitute.com

6. Booth, R (2014). *The Venus Week: Discover the Powerful Secret of Your Cycle at Any Age (Revised Edition)*. Beauty Booth LLC.

7. Griffin, E (2012, Dec 5). *What the Moon has to do with your Menstrual Cycle*. Retrieved from http://ellegriffin.com/what-the-moon-has-to-do-with-your-menstrual-cycle/

8. Griffin, E (Producer) (2014, Oct 31). The Moon and Your Menstrual Cycle Featuring Elle Griffin. Over the Moon Radio. Podcast retrieved from http://overthemoonmag.com/2014/10/the-moon-your-menstrual-cycle-featuring-elle-griffin/

9. Starkey, O (n.d.). *Cervix Throughout the Cycle*. Retrieved from http://beautifulcervix.com/your-cycle/

10. Powell, W (2014, Jan 28). *Pelvic Floor Infographic*. Retrieved from http://mutusystem.com/pelvic-floor-infographic.html

11. Chartered Society of Physiotherapy Press Release (2009, May 6). *Large numbers of men and women risk unnecessary incontinence and sexual frustration due to their ignorance and neglect of their pelvic floor muscles, say chartered physiotherapists.*

Retrieved from http://www.csp.org.uk/press-releases/2009/05/06/pelvic-floor-ignorance-leading-unnecessary-incontinence-sexual-frustration

12. Kegel, A (1952). Stress incontinence and genital relaxation; a nonsurgical method of increasing the tone of sphincters and their supporting structures. *Clinical Symposia*, 4(2), 35-51.

13. Bowman, K (2014). *Move Your DNA: Restore Your Health Through Natural Movement.* Propriometrics Press.

14. Mulligan, T (2013, Feb 4). *Posture Must Be Consistent.* Retrieved from http://www.hab-it.com/blog/posture-must-be-consistent/

15. Burrell, J (2014, Aug 24). *"Exhale on Exertion"... Why We Need to Teach the Post Natal Client to "Lift for Life!"* Retrieved from http://www.burrelleducation.com/2014/exhale-on-exertion-why-we-need-to-teach-the-post-natal-client-to-lift-for-life/

16. Bowman, K (2011). *Every Woman's Guide to Foot Pain Relief: The New Science of Healthy Feet.* BenBella Books.

17. Shafik A, El-Sibai O (2000). Levator ani muscle activity in pregnancy and the postpartum period: a myoelectric study. *Clin Exp Obstet Gynecol*, 27(2), 129-32.

18. Burrell, J. E-mail message to author, April 9, 2015.

19. Hagen, S, Stark, D, Cattermole, D (2004). A United Kingdom-wide survey of physiotherapy practice in the treatment of pelvic organ prolapse. *Physiotherapy*, 90(1), 19-26. DOI: 10.1016/S0031-9406(03)00003-8

20. Urinary Tract Infections in Adults (last updated 2013, March). In *Urology Care Foundation, The Official Foundation of the American Urological Association* online website. Retrieved from http://www.urologyhealth.org/urology/index.cfm?article=47

21. Whitlock, J (n.d.). *Questions to Ask Your Surgeon Before a Hysterectomy.* Retrieved from http://surgery.about.com/od/beforesurgery/a/QuestionsHyster.htm

22. Kinkade S (2007). Evaluation and treatment of acute low back pain. *Am Fam Physician*, 75(8), 1181-8.

23. Perina, D (2011). Mechanical back pain. *Medscape Reference.* Retrieved from http://emedicine.medscape.com

24. Subak L, et al. (2009). Weight loss to treat urinary incontinence in overweight and obese women. *N Engl J Med, 360*(5), 481-90.

25. De Pergola, G., & Silvestris, F. (2013). Obesity as a Major Risk Factor for Cancer. *Journal of Obesity*, 2013, 291546. DOI:10.1155/2013/291546

26. Dalebout, K (Producer) (2014, December 30). Dr. Joy Jacobs [Episode 61]. *The Wellness Wonderland Podcast.* Podcast retrieved from http://thewellnesswonderland.simplecast.fm/episodes/6235-061-dr-joy-jacobs

27. Denisko, Y, Smith, D (2010). *Laxatives: Proceed With Caution.* Retrieved from http://www.consumer-health.com/services/LaxativesProceedwithCaution.php

28. Andreeva, N (2014). *Happy Belly: A Woman's Guide to Feeling Vibrant, Light, and Balanced.* Advantage Media.

29. Raichur, P (1997). *Absolute Beauty: Radiant Skin and Inner Harmony Through the Ancient Secrets of Ayurveda.* HarperCollins.

30. Gaskins, A et al. (2009). Effect of daily fiber intake on reproductive function: the BioCycle Study. *The Am J of Clin Nutri*, 90(4), 1061–1069.

31. Schulz, ML (2006). *The New Feminine Brain: Developing Your Intuitive Genius*. Atria Books.

32. LaPorte, D (n.d.). *We know you're busy. Now shut up about it*. Retrieved from http://www.daniellelaporte.com/we-know-youre-busy-now-shut-up-about-it

33. Gottfried, S (2013). *The Hormone Cure: Reclaim Balance, Sleep, Sex Drive and Vitality Naturally with The Gottfried Protocol*. New York: Scribner.

34. Crawt, S (Interviewer) & Gedgaudas, N (Interviewee) (2014). *The Unconventional Weight Loss Convention, Interview with Nora Gedgaudas: The Impact Our Adrenals Stress, and What We Eat Have on Our Ability to Lose Weight* [Interview transcript]. Retrieved from The Unconventional Weight Loss Convention online website: http://unconventionalweightloss.com/order

35. Autoimmune Disease in Women (n.d.). In *American Autoimmune Related Diseases Association, Inc.* online website. Retrieved from http://www.aarda.org/autoimmune-information/autoimmune-disease-in-women

36. Prevalence and Impact of Thyroid Disease (n.d.). In *The American Thyroid Association* online website. Retrieved from http://www.thyroid.org/media-main/about-hypothyroidism/

37. Amino, N (1988). Autoimmunity and hypothyroidism. *Baillieres Clin Endocrinol Metab*, 2(3):591-617.

38. Kresser, C (n.d.). *The Most Important Thing You May Not Know About Hypothyroidism*. Retrieved from http://chriskresser.com/the-most-important-thing-you-may-not-know-about-hypothyroidism

39. Karasik, D. and Ferrari, S. L. (2008), Contribution of Gender-Specific Genetic Factors to Osteoporosis Risk. *Annals of Human Genetics*, 72(5): 696–714. DOI: 10.1111/j.1469-1809.2008.00447.x

40. Osteoporosis/Osteopenia (n.d.). In *National Women's Health Network* online website. Retrieved from http://nwhn.org/osteoporosis-osteopenia

41. Grogan, M (2013, April 19). *I've read that calcium supplements may increase the risk of heart attack. Is this true?* Retrieved from http://www.mayoclinic.org/diseases-conditions/heart-attack/expert-answers/calcium-supplements/faq-20058352

42. David, M (2005). *The Slow Down Diet: Eating for Pleasure, Energy, and Weight Loss*. Healing Arts Press.

43. Gardner, A (2008, Oct 31). Almost Half of Women Have Sexual Problems. *The Washington Post*. Retrieved from http://www.washingtonpost.com/wp-dyn/content/article/2008/10/31/AR2008103101138.html

44. Bouchez, C (2008, Nov 19). *Escape from Hormone Horrors – What You Can Do*. Retrieved from http://www.webmd.com/women/features/escape-hormone-horrors-what-you-can-do

45. Barton-Schuster, D. (n.d.). Traditional Vagina Steam for Healthy Fertility. Retrieved from http://natural-fertility-info.com/vagina-steam.html

46. Brashear (2015, Jan 9). *Why Vaginal Steaming Could Be the Best Thing We'll Try This Year*. Retrieved from http://www.elephantjournal.com/2015/01/why-vaginal-steaming-could-be-the-best-thing-well-try-this-year/

47. Herber-Gast, G & Mishra, G (2013). Fruit, Mediterranean-style, and high-fat and-sugar diets are associated with the risk of night sweats and hot flushes in midlife: results from a prospective cohort study. *Am J Clin Nutri, 97*(5): 1092-1099.

48. Endocrine Disruptors (last updated 2013, Aug 28). In *Canadian Centre for Occupational Health and Safety* online website. Retrieved from http://www.ccohs.ca/oshanswers/chemicals/endocrine.html

49. Sherburn M. Evidence for pelvic floor physical therapy in the elderly. Cited in: Shelly B, Neville C, Strauhal MJ, Jenkyns P (2010). *Pelvic Physical Therapy Level 3.* Published by the Section on Women's Health of the American Physical Therapy Association.

50. Huffington, Arianna (2014). *Thrive: The Third Metric to Redefining Success and Creating a Life of Well-Being, Wisdom, and Wonder.* Harmony.

51. Melville G, Chang D, Colagiuri B, Marshall P, Cheema B (2012). Fifteen minutes of chair-based yoga postures or guided meditation performed in the office can elicit a relaxation response. *Evidence-Based Complementary and Alternative Medicine,* Article ID 501986, 9 pages. DOI:10.1155/2012/501986.

52. Dusek J, et al. (2008) Genomic counter-stress changes induced by the relaxation response. *PLoS ONE 3*(7): e2576.

53. What is Yin Yang? (n.d.). In *Personal Tao: Always Dream Even When Awake* online website. Retrieved from http://personaltao.com/teachings/questions/what-is-yin-yang/

54. Body Balance (2006, July 11). In *DailyOM: Nurturing Mind, Body, & Spirit* online website. Retrieved from http://www.dailyom.com/articles/2006/3938.html

55. Veerman, J et al. (2012). Television viewing time and reduced life expectancy: a life table analysis. *Br J Sports Med, 46*(13): 927-930. DOI:10.1136/bjsports-2011-085662

56. Schmid, D, & Leitzmann, M (2014). Television viewing and time spent sedentary in relation to cancer risk: a meta-analysis. *JNCI J Natl Cancer Inst, 106*(7): dju098 DOI:10.1093/jnci/dju098

57. Ekeland, U et al. (2015). Physical activity and all-cause mortality across levels of overall and abdominal adiposity in European men and women: the European Prospective Investigation into Cancer and Nutrition Study (EPIC). *Am J Clin Nutr 2015 ajcn.100065*; First published online Jan 14, 2015. DOI:10.3945/ajcn.114.100065

58. Press Association (2015, Jan 14). Scientists recommend 20-minute daily walk to avoid premature death. *The Guardian.* Retrieved from http://www.theguardian.com/lifeandstyle/2015/jan/14/scientists-recommend-20-minute-daily-walk-premature-death

59. Hulme, J (2005). *Solving the Mystery of the Pelvic Rotator Cuff in Human Function and Movement: Back Pain, Balance, and Bladder Health.* Phoenix Publishing.

60. Teta, J & Teta, K (2011). *The Metabolic Effect Diet: Eat More, Work Out Less, and Actually Lose Weight While You Rest.* Harper.

61. Kelley, S (2012, Dec 19). *Let's Get Naked: Sheila Kelley at TEDx American Riviera.* Retrieved from http://tedxtalks.ted.com/video/Lets-Get-Naked-Sheila-Kelley-at

62. Caetano, A, Tavares, M, & Lopes, M (2007). Urinary incontinence and physical

activity practice. *Revista Brasileira de Medicina do Esporte,* 13(4), 270-274. Retrieved April 22, 2015 from http://www.scielo.br/scielo.php?script=sci_arttext&pid=S1517-86922007000400012&lng=en&tlng=en. 10.1590/S1517-86922007000400012.

63. Kelley, S (2003). *The S Factor: Strip Workouts for Every Woman.* Workman Publishing Company.

64. Berceli, D (2008). *The Revolutionary Trauma Release Process: Transcend Your Toughest Times.* Namaste Publishing.

65. Food Intolerance – Definition (last updated 2013, March 23). In *The Food Intolerance Institute of Australia* online website. Retrieved from http://www.foodintol.com/food-sensitivities

66. Kim, D, & Camilleri, M (2000). Serotonin: a mediator of the brain-gut connection. *The American Journal of Gastroenterology,* 95(10): 2698-2709.

67. Everything you always wanted to know about the Gut Microbiota (n.d.). In *Gut Microbiota Worldwatch: Public Information Service from European Society of Neurogastroenterology and Motility* online website. Retrieved from http://www.gutmicrobiotawatch.org/gut-microbiota-info/

68. Sanmukhani, J et al. (2014). Efficacy and safety of curcumin in major depressive disorder: a randomized controlled trial. *Phytother Res,* 28(4): 579-85. DOI: 10.1002/ptr.5025. Epub 2013 Jul 6.

69. Ruper, S (2014). *Sexy by Nature: The Whole Foods Solution to Radiant Health, Life-Long Sex Appeal, and Soaring Confidence.* Victory Belt Publishing.

70. Katz, R (2013). *The Longevity Kitchen: Satisfying, Big-Flavor Recipes Featuring the Top 16 Age-Busting Power Foods.* Ten Speed Press.

71. Drummond, J (2014). *Module 4, Webinar 1: Fertility Rituals, The Normal Pregnancy, and Preconception Support* [PowerPoint slides]. Retrieved from the Integrative Pelvic Health Institute member portal (IPHI students only): http://integrativepelvichealthinstitute.com

72. Nutt, A (2015, Jan 12). BPA alternative disrupts normal brain-cell growth, is tied to hyperactivity, study says. *The Washington Post.* Retrieved from http://www.washingtonpost.com/national/health-science/bpa-alternative-disrupts-normal-brain-cell-growth-is-tied-to-hyperactivity-study-says/2015/01/12/a9ecc37e-9a7e-11e4-a7ee-526210d665b4_story.html

73. Munro, M (2015, Jan12). Researchers advice pregnant women to limit exposure to receipts and plastic. *Canada.com* (owned and operated by Postmedia Network Inc.). Retrieved from http://o.canada.com/news/national/researchers-advise-pregnant-women-to-limit-exposure-to-receipts-and-plastic

74. Aga, M et al. (2001). Preventive effect of Coriandrum sativum (Chinese parsley) on localized lead deposition in ICR mice. *Ethnopharmacol,* 77(2-3):203-8.

75. Richard, M (2012, November 30). Best air-filtering houseplants, according to NASA. *Mother Nature Network.* Retrieved from http://www.mnn.com/health/healthy-spaces/stories/best-air-filtering-houseplants-according-to-nasa

76. Kratina, K (n.d.). Orthorexia Nervosa. *National Eating Disorders Association (NEDA)* online website. Retrieved from http://www.nationaleatingdisorders.org/orthorexia-nervosa

77. Shimoff, M (2009). *Happy for No Reason: 7 Steps to Being Happy from the Inside Out*. Atria books.

78. Rhodes, M (2014). *Heart Beats: Music Infused Insights* [audio CD]. Sounds True.

79. Hay, L (1984). *You Can Heal Your Life*. Hay House.

80. Kerr, F (n.d.). *Love Yourself*. Retrieved from http://highonclearskin.com/how-to-get-clear/love-yourself/

81. Ross, C (2012). Why Do Women Hate Their Bodies?. *Psych Central*. Retrieved from http://psychcentral.com/blog/archives/2012/06/02/why-do-women-hate-their-bodies/

82. Ruper, S (2014, Nov 12). *Six Psychological Hangups Preventing You From Having Good Sex*. Retrieved from http://paleoforwomen.com/6-psychological-hangups-preventing-you-from-having-good-sex

83. Cabeca, A (2015, February 12). Help Doctor, My Sex Drive Has No Pulse! [Webinar Recording]. Retrieved from (private access only): http://www.sexualcpr.com

84. Sacomori, C, & Cardoso, F (2015). Predictors of Improvement in Sexual Function of Women with Urinary Incontinence After Treatment with pelvic floor exercises: a secondary analysis. J of Sexual Med 2015; 12:746-755. DOI: 10.1111/jsm.12814

85. Hanh, T (1999). *The Heart of the Buddha's Teaching: Transforming Suffering into Peace, Joy, and Liberation*. Broadway Books.

86. Mercier, P (2007). *The Chakra Bible: The Definitive Guide to Chakra Energy*. Sterling.

87. Chia M, & Carlton Abrams R (2005). *The Multi-Orgasmic Woman*. Rodale.

88. Heiman J, & LoPiccolo J (1992). *Becoming Orgasmic (revised and expanded edition)*. New York: Fireside.

89. Daedone, N (2012). *Slow Sex: The Art and Craft of the Female Orgasm*. Grand Central Life & Style.

90. Dooley, M (2010). *Infinite Possibilities: The Art of Living Your Dreams*. Atria Books/Beyond Words.

91. Constine, J (2014, July 23). American Users Spend And Average of 40 Minutes Per Day on Facebook. Retrieved from http://techcrunch.com/2014/07/23/facebook-usage-time/

92. Vogel, L (2014, Dec 15). Ask Yourself This Question If You Want To Be Blissfully Happy. Retrieved from https://youtu.be/Pi6cCIQrmSU

Acknowledgements

To everyone I interviewed in the process of writing this book, thank you. Your stories have brought these pages to life.

To my editor, Libby Provost – your sensitivity and keen eye for detail helped me avoid numerous foot-in-mouth incidents and, of course, grammatical errors. I am eternally grateful for your assistance and for your friendship.

To my mentors in the "health world," particularly Jessica Drummond and everyone at the Integrative Pelvic Health Institute, and to everyone I've read, studied, and referenced in the Resources section, thank you for being an ever-fascinating source of inspiration and information.

To my business mentors, particularly Natalie Eckdahl of www.bizchix.com, thank you for your energy and consistent motivation to reach for (and achieve) more.

To my cadre of personal healers, including Eva Theiss, Linda Seelig, Amanda Brust, Kim Fun (my Compassion Dakini), Danielle Paige, and Lisa Finchum, thank you for bringing me back to me.

To my "Fem Babies," Teresa, Tara, Anna, and Amy, thanks for always supporting me and my business endeavors. I hope to build BIG things with all of you in the future.

To Beth Danowsky, with whom I bonded over sauerkraut... Thanks for your loyalty and friendship. I know we will continue to do great things together.

To Katy Kemp, the beautiful, generous soul that you are... Thank you for all of your assistance and love over the years. It's been quite a ride. I am so grateful!

For the fabulous cover design, the painstaking process of interior formatting and layout, and for your unfailing support in all things I have done and will do, THANK YOU to my dear cousin Kelly Hampson. You are such a blessing in my life.

Speaking of the cover, special thanks to Jessica Thompson of Jessica Images (www.jessicaimages.com). Your generosity is matched only by your ability to capture the exquisite beauty and essence of the women you photograph! You have a gift.

Thank you to Leah Webb Neu of Lavish Looks by Leah for making us feel pampered and beautiful during the cover shoot. **And to my cover models, you know who you are! I love you, naked ladies!**

Thank you, Lindsey White of Lindsey White Photo (www.lindseywhitephoto. com), for the clean, precise, crystal-clear images seen throughout the interior of *Lady Bits*.

A big thanks to Jen, my dear friend and the beautiful model for many of the photos.

Jessica Aiduk: Thank you for your skills, friendship, and GENEROUS support (on so many levels). Your editorial input and photographic additions helped take *Lady Bits* over the top!

Christine Niemann of Wooni Pixel (www.woonipixel.com) – thank you for your patience, time, and talent. Your videography skills blow me away, and the Inner Core Energizer videos add so much value to this book.

Thank you to Andrea Hughbanks and the staff at EveryBody Physical Therapy for giving me my start as a women's health physical therapist in Portland, Oregon.

A big shout out to my wonderful FemFusion class participants! I love your energy and enthusiasm. Thank you for giving me a platform for talking about kegels and booty circles, and thank you **from the bottom of my heart** for believing in me.

Thank you, Jenny Doyle, for giving FemFusion Fitness a start in Germany and for your generous support of me in all ways, always.

To the women who read and critiqued early drafts of this book – Ronel, Jennifer, Jessica, Katie, Tasha, Jenny, and Amy – thank you! You helped fine-tune *Lady Bits* to make it what it is today. Your assistance and collective wisdom means so much!

To Pubslush and all of the *Lady Bits* supporters, thank you for helping finance my dream! **A special shout out goes to:** Leah Ray, Sandra Larsen, Amanda Komp, Amanda Mortlock, Karen Loos, Britta Koehler, Genni Day, Rachel Anderson, Christine Ford, Ronel Van der Berg, Vanessa Moen, Alice Weyrauch, Karen Waller, Jenn Edden, Anna Henry, Cat Martin, Julia Markova, Brittany Caitlin, Cheryl DeClerque, Lisa Patmor, Jin Shin, Colleen Grogan, Cinda Helmin, John Salmon, Marcia Schulmerich, Cynthia Shafer, and Amy Lawson... Your generosity is helping me spread the *Lady Bits* message to women all over the world.

To my entire family, extended and nuclear – although we don't get to see as much of each other as I'd like, you are always in my heart. Colleen and John Grogan, you are the most generous and supportive in-laws a girl could ask for. Thank you for Chris. Thank you for YOU!

To my dear parents – thank you for helping me to become the woman that I am today. I strive to surprise you with ever-evolving ideas and ventures, and no matter how old I am, I hope to always make you proud.

To my wonderful husband and son: I can't describe how much I love you both. Thank you for lifting me up when I feel down, thank you for giving me the time and space to focus on my dreams, and thank you for being everything that I am not. I can't imagine life without you.

It's not just about looking good.

it's about

FEELING GOOD

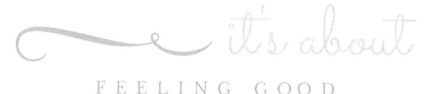

femfusionfitness
EAT CLEAN. MOVE EVERY DAY.
SHINE BRIGHTER!

About the Author

Brianne Grogan is a Doctor of Physical Therapy, an AFAA certified group fitness instructor, a certified Women's Health and Nutrition Coach (WHNC) through the Integrative Pelvic Health Institute, and the founder of FemFusion® Fitness.

An Oregon native, Brianne currently lives in Europe with her husband and son. She enjoys world travel, all things related to the great outdoors, and – of course – clean eating and moving every day. Learn more about Brianne and FemFusion® Fitness at www.femfusionfitness.com.

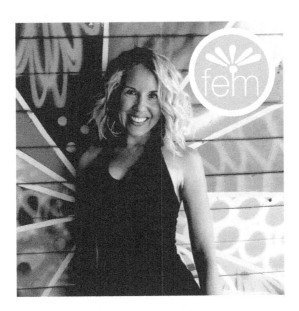